PRACTICAL PROCEDURES

IN GENE

Other titles from Scion

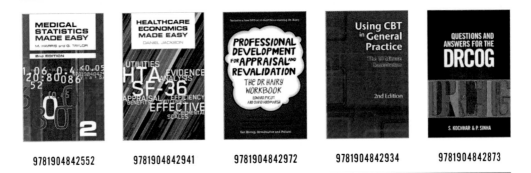

| 9781904842552 | 9781904842941 | 9781904842972 | 9781904842934 | 9781904842873 |

For more information see **www.scionpublishing.com**

PRACTICAL PROCEDURES

IN GENERAL PRACTICE

Suneeta Kochhar

MBBS, MRCGP (2010), MRCS (2007), DRCOG, DFSRH
GP in East Sussex

Scion

© Scion Publishing Ltd, 2013

ISBN 978 1 904842 996

First published in 2013

A CIP catalogue record for this book is available from the British Library.

Scion Publishing Limited
The Old Hayloft, Vantage Business Park, Bloxham Road, Banbury,
Oxfordshire OX16 9UX, UK
www.scionpublishing.com

Important Note from the Publisher

The information contained within this book was obtained by Scion Publishing Limited from sources believed by us to be reliable. However, while every effort has been made to ensure its accuracy, no responsibility for loss or injury whatsoever occasioned to any person acting or refraining from action as a result of information contained herein can be accepted by the author or publishers.

Although every effort has been made to ensure that all owners of copyright material have been acknowledged in this publication, we would be pleased to acknowledge in subsequent reprints or editions any omissions brought to our attention.

Readers should remember that medicine is a constantly evolving science and while the author and publishers have ensured that all dosages, applications and practices are based on current indications, there may be specific practices which differ between communities. You should always follow the guidelines laid down by the manufacturers of specific products and the relevant authorities in the country in which you are practising.

Line artwork by Hilary Strickland Illustration, Bath, UK
Typeset by Phoenix Photosetting, Chatham, UK
Printed by MPG Printgroup, UK

Contents

Chapter 3: Joint injections   39

Chapter 4: Steroid injections in the upper limb   47

Chapter 5: Steroid injections in the lower limb   75

Chapter 6: Long-acting reversible methods of contraception 87

Chapter 7: Other procedures   95

Preface

There is evidence in the UK that minor surgical procedures carried out by GPs in primary care have high levels of patient satisfaction and are cost-effective. As such, many GPs are looking to develop a minor surgery Directed Enhanced Service (DES), which includes joint injections and invasive procedures such as excisions. In addition, provision of long-acting reversible contraceptive methods such as Nexplanon® and Mirena® coils may also be undertaken in general practice. GPs with a special interest may wish to investigate the provision of carpal tunnel decompression, or no scalpel vasectomy; these procedures are covered in the book to indicate what is possible within general practice, though it should be noted that they are by no means routine and usually require specialist training and accreditation.

This book was written to serve as a guide and aide-memoire to the broad range of practical procedures that are routinely performed in general practice. However, it is not intended as a substitute for gaining relevant practical experience and clinicians may need to undergo appropriate additional training: the Royal College of General Practitioners offers an increasing number of minor surgery and joint injection courses. In addition, a postgraduate qualification in dermatology and/or dermatological surgery may represent a way of demonstrating structured learning.

For any practical procedure, a successful service relies on patient selection and appropriate pre-assessment as well as surgical skills, and the book provides guidance on both selection and assessment. Finally, any procedure must be undertaken in line with local guidelines to ensure that funding is provided, and the book will help you to understand when funding may be restricted.

GPs offering minor surgery and other practical procedures should be able to reduce referrals, increase practice income and provide a better service to their patients. If you are looking to develop a minor surgery DES, or simply looking to see what other practical procedures you might add to your service, then I hope that this book will help.

Suneeta Kochhar
January 2013

About the author

Suneeta Kochhar is a GP Principal at Churchwood Medical Practice in St Leonards-on-Sea, in East Sussex, where she is women's health and minor surgery lead at the practice. She completed the Membership of the Royal College of General Practitioners (MRCGP) examination in 2010 and completed the Membership of the Royal College of Surgeons (MRCS) examination in 2007. She also has the Diploma of the Royal College of Obstetricians and Gynaecologists (DRCOG) and the Diploma of the Faculty of Sexual and Reproductive Healthcare (DFSRH).

CHAPTER 1

Introduction to minor surgery

Specification for a Directed Enhanced Service in minor surgery

The specification for a DES in minor surgery should be read in detail prior to offering a minor surgery service[1], remembering that the actual content of the DES in minor surgery will be locally negotiated. The key features and requirements, based on my experience of setting up and running such a service and the DES document, are discussed below.

Cryotherapy, curettage and cauterisation may all be provided by GPs. These services are considered to be an additional part of core services under General Medical Services (GMS) or Personal Medical Services (PMS) contracts, and payment for these services is included in these contracts. As part of a DES there are two main categories for payment:

- the first category covers injections for muscles, tendons and joints – remuneration is typically in the order of £40.

- the second category covers invasive procedures such as incisions and excisions – remuneration is typically in the order of £80–90.

- a third category may include injections of varicose veins and piles, although these are not often performed in general practice.

The service specification locally will follow the principles and pricing structure of the national specification for the provision of minor surgery.

As part of a DES, under the 'injections of muscles, tendons and joints' category, the following procedures may be included as part of the service specification locally: shoulder, elbow (medial and lateral epicondylitis), carpal tunnel, trigger finger, metacarpophalangeal joints, trochanteric bursitis, knee and De Quervain's tenosynovitis. Minor surgery covered by the invasive procedures category that may be undertaken in general practice includes incision and drainage of abscesses and ingrown toenail surgery. If there are persistent symptoms and no diagnostic doubt, epidermal cysts, lipomata, pigmented skin lesions such as seborrhoeic keratoses and naevi, as well as dermatofibromas, may also be removed. Treatment for cosmetic reasons is unlikely to be funded under the DES. Basal cell carcinomas that are low risk may be removed in primary care provided that the rel-

---

[1] Full details available from 'The Primary Medical Services (Direct Enhanced Services) (England) Directions 2006' published by the Department of Health: www.dh.gov.uk/en/Publicationsandstatistics/Publications/PublicationsLegislation/DH_4136869 [last accessed 8/1/2013].

evant local accreditation process (as determined by the local Primary Care Organisation and secondary care) has been followed.

Pre-requisites for this enhanced service include:

- ensuring that those undertaking procedures have the necessary experience, skills and training; up to date resuscitation skills are important, as is the demonstration of a certain level of minor surgery activity

- regular audit, appraisal and continuing professional development

- making appropriate arrangements for infection control is an absolute requirement

- written consent should be obtained for surgical procedures

- all specimens should be sent for histological examination.

In the future it is likely that GPs newly undertaking minor surgery will have to demonstrate competency to an external body, probably using assessment tools such as Direct Observation of Procedural Skills (DOPS). Those with an existing minor surgery service are likely to have to demonstrate the same standards.

Pre-requisites

Facilities

A safe and clean environment is imperative when setting up a minor surgery service. To be adequate, the room needs to be large enough to ensure that access with an operating trolley around the couch is not an issue, and there must be access to allow for resuscitation equipment to be used in the event of an emergency. Furthermore there should be dedicated clean areas, with a sink for hand washing, and dirty areas for used equipment and swabs. National guidance is available on standards for premises[2], for example, a minor surgery room should be at least 17.5 m^2 in size and used exclusively for this purpose and/or for other treatments. Adequate lighting, ventilation and heating are important and the requirements for these may be revised in future guidance from the Care Quality Commission (CQC).

Adequate background lighting supplemented with a ceiling-mounted surgical light on a flexible arm is ideal. Additional lighting may be required if it is not possible to have a surgical light. An adjustable (height and tilting)

---

[2] Department of Health. Health building note 46: General medical practice premises

minor surgery couch is an important consideration both for comfort of the patient as well as the surgeon. The couch is ideally placed centrally in the room with space around it on all sides to accommodate an operating trolley. The couch and the operating trolley should be wiped down with antiseptic wipes between cases.

The floor should be washable, jointless and have no skirting ledge. All surfaces must be washable and be able to withstand regular chemical cleaning. Lighting must be easy to clean. The hand basin must be fitted with elbow-operated mixer taps and not be used for equipment or disposal of contaminated waste. Liquid soap and chemical hand-washing solution should be wall-hung and be elbow-operated.

Resuscitation equipment

Resuscitation equipment must be available to deal with any unexpected complications such as anaphylaxis. Equipment should include airway adjuncts, artificial ventilation, needles, syringes, intravenous cannulae and may include a defibrillation unit. Adrenaline, diazepam, chlorphenamine, hydrocortisone and oxygen should be stocked. The surgeon and any assistant should be trained in the use of resuscitation equipment. It is also important to be aware of local needlestick injury guidance.

Cautery

For most minor surgery procedures electrocautery is not necessary. Chemical cautery using, for example, aluminium chloride hexahydrate (Driclor) or phenol (50–100%) may be employed for superficial wounds; note that phenol is not recommended except for its use in ingrown toenail removal.

Requirement for an assistant

Registered nurses or Health Care Assistants (HCAs) with a level 3 NVQ qualification may provide assistance. Practice nurses assisting in minor surgery procedures should be appropriately trained and competent, taking into consideration their professional accountability and the Nursing and Midwifery Council guidelines on the scope of their professional practice.

There is no specific guidance regarding the assistant's role for minor surgery procedures except that they should be familiar with procedures and what is required of them. For example, the assistant may be vital in setting up the operating trolley, adjusting the light source and ensuring that histological specimens are appropriately labelled and despatched.

Infection control

A practice undertaking minor surgery should have an infection control policy that is compliant with guidance stipulated by the local Primary Care Organisation (PCO); for example, there may be guidance related to the use of sterile instruments or approved sterilisation procedures. Furthermore, an infection control policy will include details of the handling of excised specimens and the disposal of clinical waste.

Protective eyewear should be considered to reduce the risk of splash injuries.

Immunisation against hepatitis B is necessary for both surgeon and assistant.

Disposal of sharps and 'dirty' waste needs to be considered. All sharps used in minor surgery need to be accounted for and thrown in designated sharps boxes. Clinical waste and clean waste bins must be available.

Where possible, disposable sterile surgical equipment should be used to remove the need for sterilisation. If autoclaves are used for sterilisation, local guidance should be taken into consideration. If diathermy is being used for minor surgery, tips should be single use and disposable.

The risk of infection from the surgeon and their assistant may be minimised by ensuring good hand washing and sterile field techniques. Moreover, knowledge of the management of needlestick injuries and local guidance for these is important. Intraoperative techniques to achieve haemostasis and remove devitalised tissue may also minimise the risk of infection.

Patient factors may be minimised by adequate pre-operative skin preparation and advice regarding post-operative care.

Having a safe and clean environment reduces the risk of infection. There should be dedicated clean areas, with a sink for hand washing, and dirty areas for used equipment and swabs. All surfaces including the floor should be washable and be able to withstand regular chemical cleaning. Hand basins must be fitted with elbow-operated mixer taps and not be used for equipment or disposal of contaminated waste. Liquid soap and chemical hand-washing solution should be wall-hung and be elbow-operated to minimise the risk of infection.

Assessing suitability for minor surgery

Minor surgery should not be carried out if there is any diagnostic uncertainty.

Clinical history taking, skin examination, identification of skin lesions and then a decision on appropriate management, be it operative or non-operative, is important (see *Fig. 1.1*). For example, undertaking a minor surgery procedure in a patient with poorly controlled diabetes and peripheral vascular disease may not be appropriate because the risks probably outweigh the benefits. Furthermore, those who are on long-term steroids or who are immunocompromised may not be the best candidates for minor surgery due to the risk of infection and poor wound healing.

The clinical necessity for removal of a skin lesion also needs to be considered; for example, it may be appropriate to remove a skin lesion that is prone to repeated trauma and/or is symptomatic, whereas it may not be appropriate to remove a skin lesion purely for cosmetic reasons. Indeed if a skin lesion is excised for cosmetic reasons, replacing it with a scar may also be unacceptable; for example, removal of a benign skin lesion from the anterior chest wall in a female patient may result in a hypertrophic or keloid scar, and, in an elderly woman with a skin lesion to the anterior leg that has been excised, healing may be difficult and ulceration is a recognised complication. Patients should be advised that all minor surgery will produce a scar and that such a resultant scar is likely to be greater in size than the skin lesion being removed, when allowance has been made for wound closure.

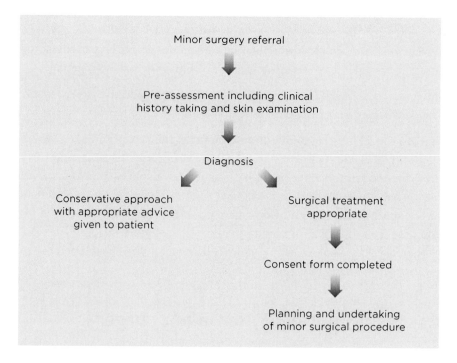

Figure 1.1: Flowchart to show summary of patient pathway.

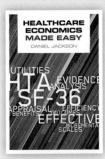
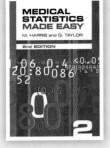
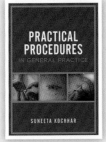
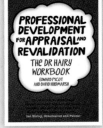
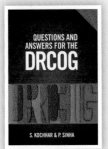
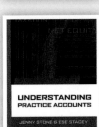

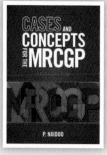
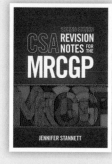
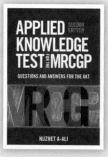
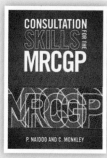

Criteria for minor surgery should also be established according to level of competence. It is recommended that operating in the mid-face should be avoided unless the surgeon has the relevant skills to obtain a good cosmetic result. For example, wound closure at the vermilion border of the lip is best undertaken by a specialist in secondary care.

Once due consideration has been given to the appropriateness of a minor surgical procedure, patients should be told what will happen on the day of the operation and informed consent obtained (see *Appendix 1: Consent to minor surgery form*). It is also useful to give the patient a simple information leaflet as an adjunct (see *Appendix 2: Patient information leaflet*).

Patients should be counselled on the risks and benefits of a procedure and procedures should be carried out with informed consent. Discussing risk involves highlighting possible risks of complications such as infection, bleeding, nerve damage and scarring.

As part of pre-assessment, a drug history should be taken; aspirin, clopidogrel and warfarin may make it difficult for haemostasis to be achieved intra-operatively. Moreover, it may be acceptable in some situations to stop warfarin pre-operatively (for example, in a case of lone atrial fibrillation), but it would be unacceptable to stop it in a patient with a metallic heart valve; an International Normalised Ratio (INR) <2 would be appropriate for most minor surgery. Aspirin and clopidogrel do not normally need to be stopped prior to minor surgery, although patients should be made aware that they are potentially more likely to bleed intra-operatively and bruise post-operatively.

Patients should also be counselled about post-operative care; it is useful to provide a leaflet for the patient to take home (see *Appendix 2: Patient information leaflet*).

Advice should be given regarding timing of suture removal. Advice should also be given about the signs of infection, to encourage patients to re-attend if they notice any early signs of this complication. Post-operatively it is recommended that surgical incisions are covered for 48 hours but that patients may safely shower after this. Immediate post-operative pain is not usually an issue because the local anaesthetic may still be effective for up to 2 hours. Patients can be advised that simple analgesia may be taken post-operatively. Advice should be given that a small amount of oozing from a wound is normal and that if there is a small amount of bleeding, this can be controlled with direct pressure. However, patients should be advised to re-attend if there is persistent blood loss or any wound concerns. Some bruising surrounding the wound may be normal.

Consent

Valid consent involves communicating effectively with patients, checking that patients can retain information, ensuring understanding, and then a valid indication of consent from the patient. In addition, advising about risks and benefits of an intervention and making a shared decision forms part of the consent process. The aforementioned criteria require the patient to have capacity to make decisions; another pre-requisite would be that consent is given voluntarily. As part of the process of providing information, the patient should be told about the implications of a procedure not being carried out. For the purposes of practical procedures undertaken in general practice, the process should be documented.

Consent forms may be downloaded from the Department of Health website[3]. In general practice, consent form 1 for 'Patient agreement to investigation or treatment' is the most appropriate and includes documentation regarding risks and benefits of a procedure. In my practice I use pre-printed consent forms (see *Appendix 1: Consent to minor surgery form*) that include documentation of risks and benefits. Intended benefits may include removal of skin lesion and therefore relief of symptoms and, by sending all specimens that are removed for histology, obtaining an accurate diagnosis. Risks of minor surgery include pain, infection, bleeding, wound breakdown, need for further treatment, risk of recurrence, need for referral to secondary care, damage to nerves and blood vessels, in addition to a reaction to local anaesthesia.

Audit

Audit of minor surgical experience is an important part of the minor surgery enhanced service and should highlight complication rates and possibly identify further areas of training or experience required. An audit record may log a patient identifier, the procedure carried out, the working diagnosis and the subsequent histological diagnosis, as well as possible complications. The audit record is created by the surgeon but should be accessible by others at practice level.

Clinical and histological outcomes should both be recorded to assess diagnostic accuracy. To this end, when histological specimens are sent, the site of the skin lesion and provisional diagnosis should be recorded. Keeping a log of activity is important and procedures should be in place to confirm that histology results have been received and action taken if necessary. It

---

[3] www.dh.gov.uk/en/Publichealth/Scientificdevelopmentgeneticsandbioethics/Consent/Consentgeneralinformation/DH_4015950 [last accessed 8/1/2013]

is recommended that histological examination is arranged for all removed material; there may be unexpected findings on histological examination which necessitate a referral to secondary care or the seeking of further advice. There must be a procedure in place for letting patients know if this is the case.

Competence

Competence in performing minor surgery may be demonstrated through training, continuing professional development, audit, and skills observation, and such evidence is required to demonstrate fitness to practise. Attendance at a multi-disciplinary team meeting to discuss histology is not required unless an appropriately trained GP performs procedures involving low risk malignancies such as basal cell carcinomas.

Current guidance from the Primary Care Commissioning website[4] advises that GPs must demonstrate that they undertake regular skin surgery sessions: a minimum of 20 surgical lists per year, with an average of 5 cases per list that are predominantly elliptical excisions. The guidance suggests that if fewer than 100 procedures are performed per year then the practitioner may demonstrate competency by undergoing further assessments.

Skin preparation

According to NICE guidance (2008, CG74: *Prevention and treatment of surgical site infection*), hair removal is not routinely recommended, although electrical clippers may be used. The most appropriate pre-operative skin preparations are aqueous chlorhexidine and povidone-iodine. NICE recommends the use of sterile gloves.

Skin marking with a single use, pre-sterilised pen *prior* to administration of local anaesthesia is advisable as part of planning a procedure, because administering local anaesthesia is likely to distort the tissue. Skin marking is carried out after taking into account cosmetic factors such as skin tension lines (see *Fig. 1.10* and *Surgical techniques* section below for further details). Furthermore, if a skin lesion is being removed adequate margins may be important, although only procedures on benign skin lesions should be carried out in primary care unless specialist training has been undertaken.

---

[4] 'Revised guidance and competences for the provision of services using GPs with Special Interests (GPwSIs) – Dermatology and skin surgery' can be accessed from: www.pcc-cic.org.uk/sites/default/files/articles/attachments/revised_guidance_and_competences_for_the_provision_of_services_using_gps_with_special_interests_0.pdf [last accessed 8/1/2013]

Setting up a sterile field to reduce the risk of infection involves:

- opening an operating pack using a 'no-touch' technique
- hand washing and putting on sterile gloves
- cleaning the operating field
- application of sterile drapes.

An assistant may not be required to help set up the sterile field, but may be important in providing further equipment if needed during the procedure using a 'no-touch' technique. This means that the surgeon should not touch areas outside the prepared sterile area and the assistant should not touch the area inside the sterile field. 'Gloving-up' also involves a 'no-touch' technique, such that gloves are opened onto a sterile surgical pack and the surgeon only touches the inside of the gloves whilst putting them on.

Local anaesthesia

Local anaesthetics work by blocking sodium channels which decreases the rate and degree of depolarisation of nerve cell membranes and so electrical impulses are not conducted. Most local anaesthetics cause vasodilatation. It is worth being aware that local anaesthetic injected into inflamed tissue, as in the case of infected epidermal cysts or abscesses, is less effective because the tissues are more acidic. Furthermore, if an excision of an epidermal cyst is to be carried out, injecting local anaesthetic into the cyst should be avoided because the resultant increase in pressure inside the cyst creates a risk of rupture.

There are three methods of administering local anaesthetic and these are described below.

Injection

Local anaesthetic may be injected into the deep dermis of the skin or the subcutaneous fat layer. Prior to injecting local anaesthetic, aspiration should be carried out to avoid inadvertent injection into a blood vessel. As mentioned earlier, the skin lesion should be marked prior to using local anaesthesia because the anaesthetic will cause some tissue distortion.

Local anaesthetics vary in their potency and duration of action. The most commonly used local anaesthetic for minor surgery is lidocaine because it has a rapid onset (compared to the slower onset bupivacaine) and the effect may last for up to a couple of hours. It may also be used in conjunction with adrenaline (for example, in a 1:200000 solution); this increases the duration of action and, due to the vasoconstrictive effects of adrenaline, may be helpful in keeping a bloodless operating field. The addition of adrenaline delays absorption which allows the maximum recommended dose of lidocaine to be increased from 3 mg/kg to 5 mg/kg (for reference, a 1% solution of lidocaine reflects a concentration of 10 mg/ml). Local anaesthetic with adrenaline is not advised for areas supplied by end arteries, such as digits.

Bupivacaine has a slower onset of action with a longer duration of block, and so for quick minor surgical procedures lidocaine is preferable.

Field block

Field block may be used as an alternative to local infiltration; this is where an area incorporating the skin lesion is anaesthetised. This involves fanning the needle under the skin to infiltrate a larger area without needing to pierce the skin again. A digital nerve block may be helpful, dependent on the type of surgery being considered. This may involve block of the volar and dorsal digital nerves at the base of a finger by injecting local anaesthetic into the web space between fingers (*Fig. 1.2*).

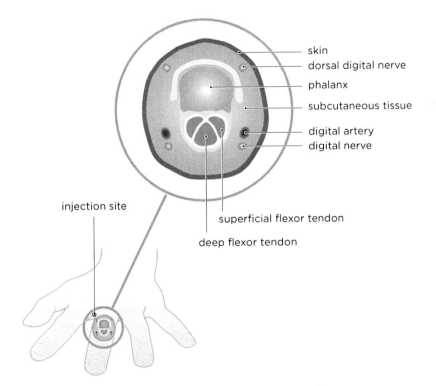

Figure 1.2: Digital nerve block of the volar and dorsal digital nerves.

Topical application

EMLA® (eutectic mixture of local anaesthetics) cream may be used as a topical application. However, because it is less efficacious it is not often used.

Adverse effects

The patient should be monitored for signs of local anaesthetic toxicity, including light-headedness, circumoral paraesthesia, and twitching.

Surgical equipment

The minimum requirements for equipment for minor surgical procedures are as follows:

- Minor surgery packs (*Figs 1.3* and *1.4*) will typically contain scissors with straight or curved blades for cutting sutures, cutting tissue and undermining.

- Scalpels with a no. 15 blade are most commonly used for skin surgery (*Fig. 1.5*), but a no. 10 blade may be useful for less fine work or for shave excisions. Cutting should be undertaken with the belly of the blade.

- Tissue forceps may be used to hold specimens and to hold wound edges; alternatively a skin hook may be used to handle wound edges (*Fig. 1.6*).

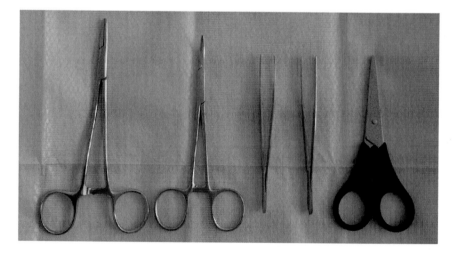

Figure 1.3: Contents of a basic minor surgery pack.
From left to right: Kilner needle holder, curved Halstead mosquito forceps, Iris toothed dissecting forceps, Iris non-toothed dissecting forceps, sharp dressing scissors.

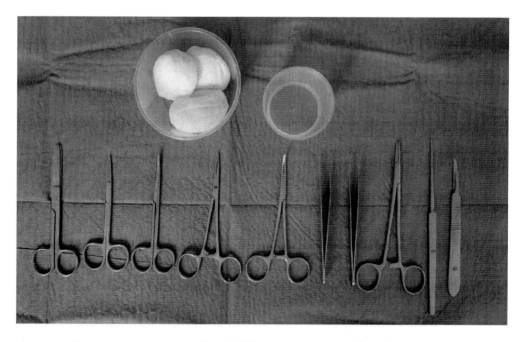

Figure 1.4: Larger minor surgery pack containing a greater range of equipment. *From left to right:* dressing scissors, Iris straight scissors, Strabismus curved blunt scissors, straight Halstead mosquito artery forceps, curved Halstead mosquito artery forceps, Adson non-toothed dissecting forceps, Adson toothed dissecting forceps, Kilner needle holder, Gillies skin hook retractor, scalpel with blade.

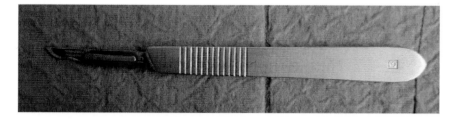

Figure 1.5: Scalpel with a no. 15 blade.

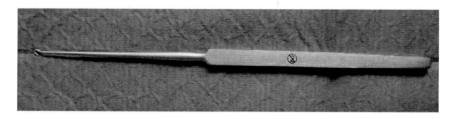

Figure 1.6: Gillies skin hook.

- Toothed forceps (*Fig. 1.7*) are recommended when handling tissue because they can offer a better grip and they avoid crushing tissue.

- Other surgical equipment includes skin punches for biopsies, needle holders (*Fig. 1.8*), artery forceps (useful in case of excessive bleeding, *Fig. 1.9*) and curettes.

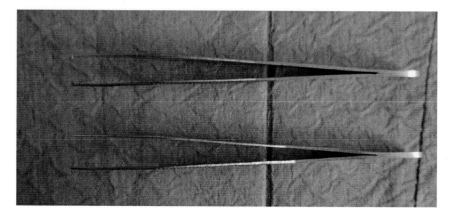

Figure 1.7: Adson toothed dissecting forceps (top) and Adson non-toothed dissecting forceps (bottom).

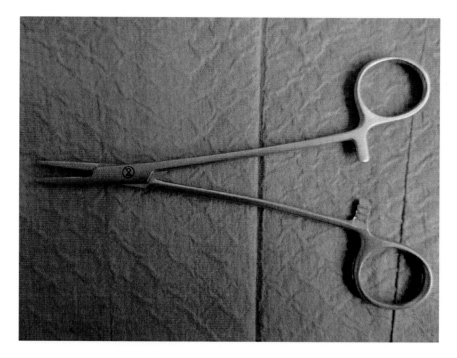

Figure 1.8: Lawrence needle holder.

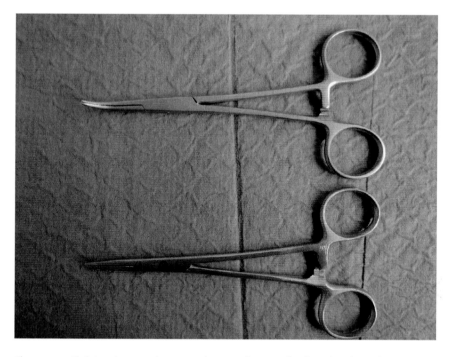

Figure 1.9: Halstead mosquito curved artery forceps (top) and Halstead mosquito straight artery forceps (bottom).

A disposable minor surgery pack suitable for the majority of minor surgical procedures in general practice may contain a wider range of equipment: self-adhesive drapes and sterile field drape, non-woven swabs, towels, gallipots, dressing scissors, Kilner needle holder, Gillies skin hook retractor, Adson toothed and non-toothed dissecting forceps, straight and curved Halstead mosquito forceps, Iris scissors, Strabismus scissors, scalpel and blade.

Sutures

Sutures may be:

- absorbable, for use in the subcutaneous layer of wounds (the most common examples are Vicryl® and PDS (polydioxanone sutures), or

- non-absorbable, which are used to approximate wounds (the most common examples are Ethilon® and Prolene®).

Sutures are usually mounted on a reverse-cutting curved needle and are sized based on their cross-section, with 5-0 being a finer suture than 4-0.

Monofilament sutures such as Ethilon® and Prolene® have a smooth surface but are more difficult to handle and knot, whereas multifilament sutures (such as Vicryl®) handle better but may harbour bacteria. A 5-0 or 6-0 suture is often used for the face and 4-0 may be used on the upper limb.

Sutures should be removed at 5–7 days from the head and neck area, at 10 days in the upper limb and trunk area, and at 14 days from the lower limbs. If the timing for suture removal is exceeded, there is an increased risk of wound infection and a 'laddered' scar may result, where there is a scar across the wound caused by the suture as well as puncture scars.

Post-operative review is often delegated to a practice nurse when the patient attends for suture removal. However, review by the doctor who performed the minor surgery may be necessary if it was felt at the time of surgery there was a complication or there were specific concerns about healing. Sometimes a patient may be reviewed to assess a particular intra-operative technique or intervention.

Surgical techniques

Wounds for minor surgery should be planned along skin tension lines (*Fig. 1.10*). This allows for the least amount of tension across a wound which aids wound approximation, and helps improve the cosmetic appearance. Wrinkling of the skin occurs when the skin is pinched across lines of maximum skin tension and so skin tension lines may be assessed by compression.

Shave excisions and curettage may be less invasive alternatives when compared to incisions or excisions; shave excisions may well be appropriate for some skin lesions. Because they are less invasive, shave excisions and curettage may produce a more favourable cosmetic result with less scarring. This is because the dermal–epidermal junction is not breached and healing by secondary intention effectively takes place.

Wound closure is a technique that requires practice and so often improves with experience. Techniques may be practised in a minor surgery course. It is important to evert the wound edges when suturing so that the dermis is opposed; where this may be difficult to achieve, mattress sutures may be helpful.

Simple interrupted suture

Most wounds may be closed using evenly placed simple interrupted sutures (*Figs 1.11* and *1.12*). This may require pre-planning in some cases (by mark-

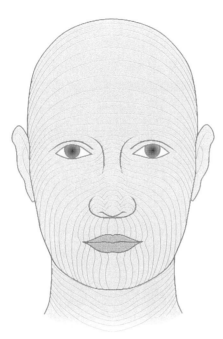

Figure 1.10: Skin tension lines of the head and neck.
Adapted from *The Merck Manual of Diagnosis and Therapy*. © 2013 by
Merck Sharp & Dohme Corp., a subsidiary of Merck & Co. Inc. Available at
www.merckmanuals.com/professional/index.html [accessed 20 Feb 2013].

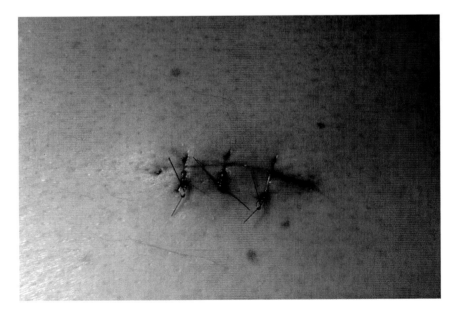

Figure 1.11: Simple interrupted Ethilon® sutures with knots laid to one side.

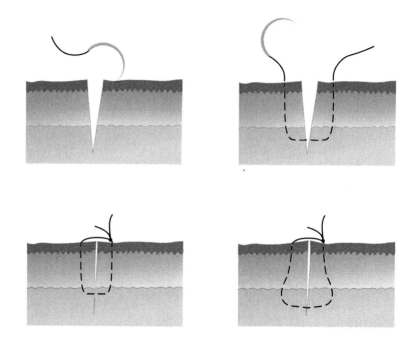

Figure 1.12: Simple interrupted suture showing the location of the suture within the skin.

ing cross-reference points on the skin prior to the incision). Alternatively the wound may be closed using a halving technique, which involves placing a suture in the centre of the wound and then successively closing the wound by dividing the wound into halves.

The middle third of a curved reverse-cutting needle should be gripped in a needle holder. A reverse-cutting needle penetrates the skin well but it is unlikely to 'cut out' (cause tearing) if used on friable tissue. One edge of the wound should be slightly everted and the needle advanced at 90° using the curve of the needle to avoid bending the needle. The opposite end of the wound is then everted and the needle passed in a similar way through the epidermis and the full thickness of the dermis. Both sides of the stitch should be symmetrical in terms of depth and width. Moreover, the stitch is wider at the base than it is superficially – this encourages wound eversion. The suture material is pulled through and tied using a square knot. The long end of the suture is wrapped around the tip of the closed needle holder twice before the shorter end of the suture is pulled with the needle holder. The initial throw of the suture is double (clockwise) and opposes the wound edges; the second is a single throw opposite to the initial one (anticlockwise). This creates a reef knot; it is this second throw that determines the tension across the wound. The final throw is single (clockwise) and the final knot is laid to one side of the wound to reduce the risk of infection.

Intradermal suture

Tension across a wound may be reduced using a buried intradermal suture (*Fig. 1.13*); this is achieved using an absorbable suture. This type of suture largely approximates the wound edges and care must be taken that it is placed evenly. If there is too much tension across a wound there is a risk of dehiscence when the scar is at its weakest, between 2 and 3 weeks after a procedure. Therefore if a deep dermal suture is in place, wound dehiscence is less likely when superficial non-absorbable sutures have been removed.

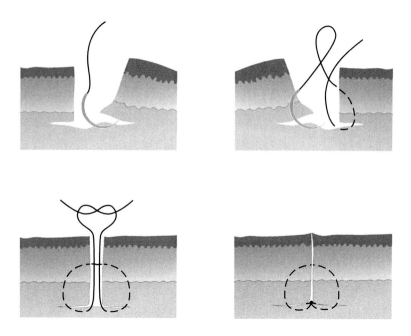

Figure 1.13: Intradermal suture.

Running suture

A running or continuous suture (*Fig. 1.14*) can also be used, although when the running suture is locked (by hooking the needle, as it emerges from the skin, under the previous loop), care must be taken not to place the wound under tension. The risk of suture marks can be minimised by using a running subcuticular suture; a non-absorbable monofilament suture such as Prolene® may be used for this purpose. A running suture is used to oppose the dermal layer where there is little skin tension.

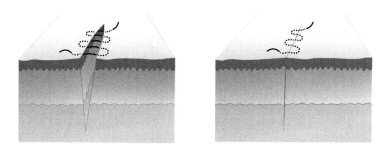

Figure 1.14: Continuous suture.

Mattress sutures

A buried intradermal (*Fig. 1.13*), or deep dermal suture, or a vertical mattress suture may be used to close a defect or eradicate dead space in a wound; this minimises the risk of infection by preventing haematoma development. A vertical mattress suture will evert skin edges, which may be useful in areas where there is laxity of the skin. It may be helpful to use a vertical mattress suture where an intradermal suture is not possible because the tissue is too friable.

A vertical mattress suture (*Fig. 1.15*) is a widely placed simple interrupted stitch followed by a more superficial stitch that is closer to the wound itself in the opposite direction. This means that the skin is punctured twice on either side of the wound.

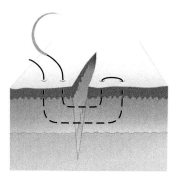

Figure 1.15: Vertical mattress suture.

A horizontal mattress suture (*Fig. 1.16*) is created by passing the suture deep in the dermis to the opposite side of the suture line and exiting the skin equidistant from the wound edge, as shown.

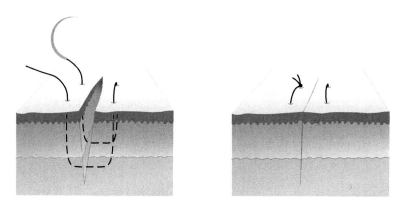

Figure 1.16: Horizontal mattress suture.

Suture removal

When removing sutures, they should be gently elevated with forceps to allow one side of the suture to be cut. The suture is grasped by the knot and gently pulled towards the wound line, i.e. vertical pressure is not exerted on the wound. A continuous subcuticular suture requires application of counter-traction on the wound when removing sutures. If additional wound support is required after suture removal, Steri-Strips™ may be considered.

Complications

Scarring is common, but can be minimised by avoiding crushing the skin edges whilst handling tissue. Hypertrophic scarring typically affects the upper chest wall with some patients being more susceptible to developing this complication. Everting wound edges and avoiding wound tension may reduce the risk of hypertrophic scarring, but patients should be advised that this complication may still occur. There is an increased risk of keloid scarring in darker skin and on the upper chest. The risk of keloid scarring may be reduced by avoiding wound tension. Creating scar tissue may result in Köebnerisation in skin conditions such as psoriasis and lichen planus.

There is a low risk of infection with minor surgery procedures; however, the risk may be higher in incision and drainage of abscesses. In the latter, wound care with the practice nurse, closure by secondary intention and possibly prophylactic antibiotics should be considered.

Bleeding intra-operatively may be controlled by direct pressure or tying off a bleeding vessel. If electrocautery is available this may be used. If post-operative bleeding occurs, pressure may be helpful. A haematoma that forms post-operatively should be addressed by achieving good haemostasis; wound exploration may be required.

Cutaneous nerve damage is inevitable but is usually not noticed due to overlapping sensory innervations. With careful assessment and patient selection, other nerve damage is unlikely to result. Care must be taken to preserve nerves and blood vessels, particularly in the head and neck area.

If there is early wound breakdown, re-suturing may be considered; however, if this occurs later in healing, closure by secondary intention may be more appropriate. When assessing patients pre-operatively an assessment is made of the probability of good healing; for example, it can be anticipated that closure is likely to be difficult in an elderly lady with a skin lesion to be excised from the anterior leg.

CHAPTER 2

Operative procedures
in minor surgery

Incision and drainage of abscesses

Incision and drainage of abscesses may be carried out in the primary care setting, depending on the area affected and clinical experience of the surgeon. Abscesses may be found in the axillae, on the back or on limbs. Antibiotic therapy alone is insufficient to treat a loculated collection of infected material. Very large or deep abscesses in areas where local anaesthesia may be difficult must be referred to secondary care so that further management may be carried out under general anaesthesia.

Procedure for incision and drainage of abscess

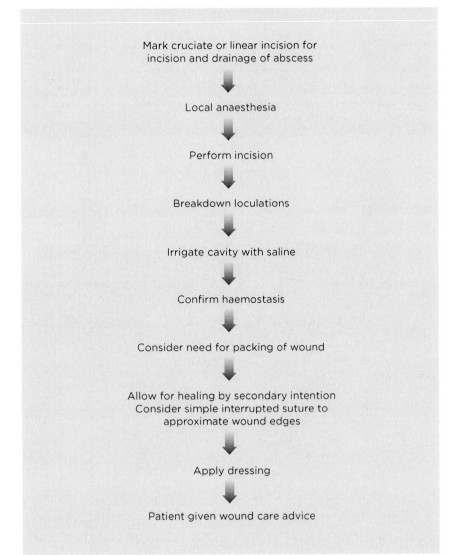

Mark cruciate or linear incision for
incision and drainage of abscess

↓

Local anaesthesia

↓

Perform incision

↓

Breakdown loculations

↓

Irrigate cavity with saline

↓

Confirm haemostasis

↓

Consider need for packing of wound

↓

Allow for healing by secondary intention
Consider simple interrupted suture to
approximate wound edges

↓

Apply dressing

↓

Patient given wound care advice

Aftercare

Suture removal at appropriate time interval if necessary, and wound review by clinician to assess healing may be carried out.

Hints and tips

- A linear incision may be used, but often a cruciate incision needs to be considered to allow pus to drain and to allow the surgeon to break down any loculations. If the loculations are not broken down, there is an increased risk of recurrence.

- After loculations have been broken down, the remaining cavity should be irrigated with saline.

- The abscess may require de-roofing and a swab may need to be sent for microbiology.

- For smaller abscesses, healing by secondary intention is usual to allow ongoing drainage from the abscess site; however, packing of the wound may need to be considered.

- Incision and drainage of an abscess usually leads to its resolution without the need for additional antibiotics.

Excision of epidermal cysts

Removal of epidermal cysts forms a significant part of a minor surgery service. These frequently occur in the head and neck region (*Fig. 2.1*) and also on the trunk. They may arise due to implantation of epidermal elements in the dermis or blockage in pilosebaceous units of the skin. They are generally benign skin lesions. An epidermal cyst is diagnosed clinically and has a typical appearance, often with a punctum. The cysts are usually asymptomatic but sometimes patients may report a smelly 'cheese-like' discharge. Epidermal cysts are often removed (*Fig. 2.2*) if they have significantly increased in size and are causing pressure symptoms. Patients often present when they have experienced recurrent infections of their epidermal cyst.

Procedure for excision of epidermal cyst

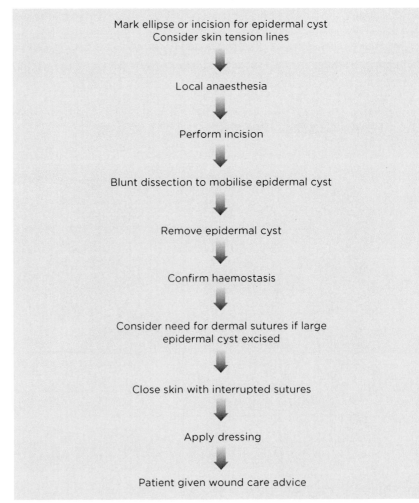

Mark ellipse or incision for epidermal cyst
Consider skin tension lines

Local anaesthesia

Perform incision

Blunt dissection to mobilise epidermal cyst

Remove epidermal cyst

Confirm haemostasis

Consider need for dermal sutures if large
epidermal cyst excised

Close skin with interrupted sutures

Apply dressing

Patient given wound care advice

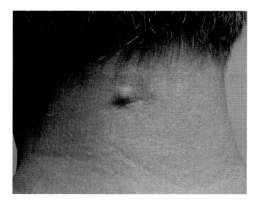
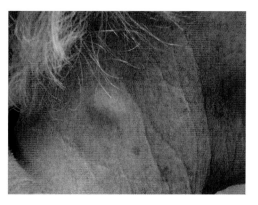

Figure 2.1: Epidermal cysts of the neck.

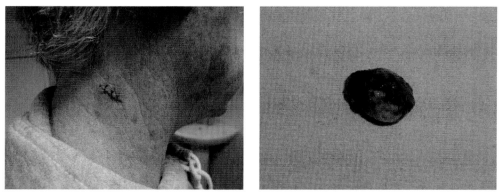

(a)   (b)

Figure 2.2: (a) Site of epidermal cyst excision; wound closure with interrupted sutures, and (b) epidermal cyst removed in its entirety.

Aftercare

Suture removal at appropriate time interval dependent on operative site.

Hints and tips

- If a patient does present with an inflamed epidermal cyst, surgery should be postponed for 6 weeks to give surgery the best chance of success. Excision of an inflamed cyst is technically more difficult because the cyst wall is likely to be more friable and therefore the cyst is more liable to rupture. However, an incision and drainage procedure may need to be carried out if an abscess has formed. This helps with resolution of the infection but does not remove the epidermal cyst itself. If an infected epidermal cyst is not incised it will eventually rupture.

- When anaesthetising the skin prior to excision of an epidermal cyst, care must be taken to avoid cyst rupture. The risk of rupture is minimised using a field block approach. An epidermal cyst may be excised through a linear incision, unless the cyst is large. In the case of larger cysts an elliptical excision that includes the punctum of the cyst is often used to avoid excess skin remaining after excision has taken place. If there is significant scar tissue an elliptical excision may also need to be considered.

- After incision, the cyst should be mobilised from the surrounding tissue, ideally avoiding rupture of its capsule and preventing release of the contents of the cyst into the wound (important to reduce the risk of recurrence). This may be achieved using blunt dissection with artery forceps and dissecting scissors. If the cyst ruptures, clamping the hole may prevent the cyst contents from emptying into the wound.

- There may be a cavity left in the skin depending on the size of the cyst removed; a deep dermal stitch may be required to close the dead space and this reduces the risk of subsequent infection. The skin is closed using simple interrupted sutures.

- A trephine excision, where the cyst contents are expressed and then the cyst wall is removed, is another option. While this method may produce a cosmetically superior result, it has a significantly increased risk of cyst recurrence and so is not generally used.

Excision of lipomas

A lipoma is a slowly growing, benign swelling that arises in the subcutaneous tissue and comprises adipose tissue. Lipomas are common and tend to develop in adulthood. They often arise on the trunk and the limbs. The aetiology is unknown; however, it is thought that trauma may sometimes be a relevant factor. Solitary lipomas are more common in women and lipomatosis is more common in men. Rarely, lipomas may be associated

Procedure for excision of lipoma

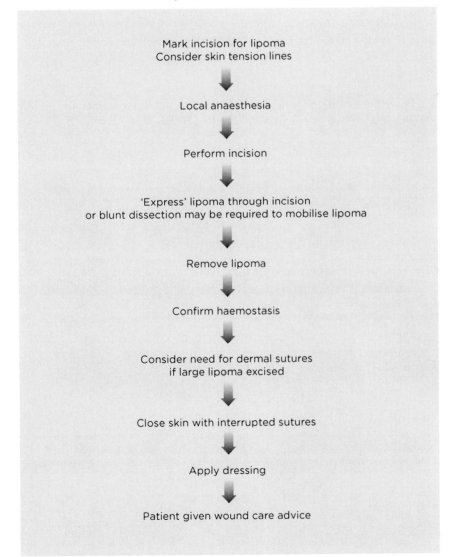

Mark incision for lipoma
Consider skin tension lines

Local anaesthesia

Perform incision

'Express' lipoma through incision
or blunt dissection may be required to mobilise lipoma

Remove lipoma

Confirm haemostasis

Consider need for dermal sutures
if large lipoma excised

Close skin with interrupted sutures

Apply dressing

Patient given wound care advice

with syndromes such as hereditary multiple lipomatosis and Gardner's syndrome (adenomatous polyps of the gastrointestinal tract, desmoid tumours, epidermoid cysts, lipomas).

Procedure for excision of lipoma

Cutaneous lipomas may be large; they are lobulated, are mobile under the skin and feel soft. Most lipomas are asymptomatic and those that are painful may be angiolipomas. Lipomas may interfere with movement, depending on their size and location. Liposarcoma rarely arises in the skin.

Aftercare

Suture removal at appropriate time interval depending on operative site.

Hints and tips

- It is often useful to mark the skin to outline the lipoma initially, to fully assess size.

- Lipomas may be excised using a linear incision because they can often be 'expressed' through this, but on occasion blunt dissection may be required. When some of the lipoma has been dissected from the surrounding tissue, artery forceps may be attached to provide traction for removal of the rest of the growth. Once dissection is complete, the lipoma is generally removed in its entirety.

- Excision of a lipoma may be associated with bleeding and tying off a small blood vessel may be necessary if electrocautery is not available.

- There may be a cavity left in the skin depending on the size of the lipoma removed; a deep dermal stitch may be required to close the dead space to reduce the risk of subsequent infection.

- The skin is usually closed using simple interrupted sutures.

Excision of pigmented skin lesions: seborrhoeic keratoses and naevi

Seborrhoeic keratoses have a typical 'stuck on' appearance and a well defined border, and they usually have plugs or pits on their surface. These may become inflamed with repeated trauma or friction. Curettage is the preferred procedure for removal of seborrhoeic keratosis; however, for particularly large or adherent keratoses, excision may be considered.

Procedure for elliptical excisions of pigmented skin lesions

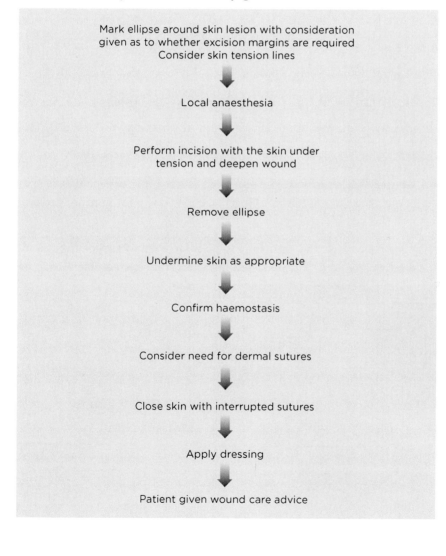

Aftercare

Suture removal at appropriate time interval depending on operative site.

Hints and tips

- Curettage is the preferred option for removal because it is less invasive and results in less scarring.

- If an elliptical excision of a pigmented skin lesion such as a seborrhoeic keratosis or a raised naevus is to be carried out, it is important to plan the incision taking into account skin tension lines and an appropriate excision margin.

- The ellipse should be marked with a 2.5–3:1 ratio to aid closure. After the area has been anaesthetised, an incision should be made with the skin under tension and the wound should then be deepened. The ellipse is then removed by cutting through the subcuticular fat, leaving a flat base and a wound with straight sides.

- To minimise skin tension it is likely that undermining or separating the dermis from the fat layer will be needed.

- Dermal sutures may still be required if there is concern about the skin being placed under tension. Good haemostasis and wound approximation should be achieved.

- Sometimes a partial closure may be performed to reduce the risk of placing a wound under tension; however, the scar produced will be wider as it will heal by secondary intention.

Basal cell carcinoma in primary care

Suspected skin cancers including high risk basal cell carcinomas, squamous cell carcinomas and malignant melanomas should be referred to secondary care. Low risk basal cell carcinomas may be managed in the community; however, multi-disciplinary team attendance is mandatory for clinicians dealing with skin cancers. Basal cell carcinomas that are low risk may be removed in primary care provided that the relevant local accreditation process (as determined by the local Primary Care Organisation and secondary care) has been followed. Current guidance is available from the Primary Care Commissioning website[1].

Morphoeic or infiltrative, as well as recurrent or persistent, basal cell carcinomas should be referred to secondary care. Referral should also be considered if primary closure after excision is likely to be difficult or where a plastic surgery opinion may be warranted. If the patient is 24 years of age or under, immunosuppressed, has Gorlin's syndrome, if the basal cell carcinoma is in the head and neck area, or if it is more than 1 cm in diameter, a referral to secondary care is essential (NICE 2006, 2010).

---

[1] 'Revised guidance and competences for the provision of services using GPs with Special Interests (GPwSIs) – Dermatology and skin surgery' can be accessed from: www.pcc-cic.org.uk/sites/default/files/articles/attachments/revised_guidance_and_competences_for_the_provision_of_services_using_gps_with_special_interests_0.pdf [last accessed 8/1/2013].

Ingrown toenails

Ingrown toenails usually affect the great toes and may cause symptoms related to inflammation and recurrent infections at the medial and/or lateral nail folds. Ingrown toenails may be related to poor nail cutting technique and poorly fitting footwear, as well as trauma. The majority of patients may be managed conservatively; for example, with antibiotic treatment and possibly silver nitrate cauterisation of granulation tissue. Hygiene measures and cotton wick insertion in the lateral groove of the nail are helpful. Surgery for ingrown toenails may be carried out in primary care, but specialist referral may be needed in patients that have diabetes, peripheral neuropathy and/or peripheral vascular disease.

The toe may be anaesthetised using a ring block (digital nerve block) and then a tourniquet applied to the base of the digit. The nail is then separated from the nail bed and avulsed using a twisting pulling action. Granulation tissue may need to be excised from the nail fold. After the tourniquet is removed, direct pressure should be applied to the nail bed prior to applying dressings.

Procedure for removal of ingrown toenail

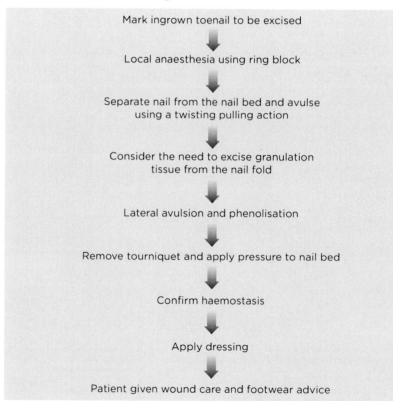

Mark ingrown toenail to be excised

Local anaesthesia using ring block

Separate nail from the nail bed and avulse using a twisting pulling action

Consider the need to excise granulation tissue from the nail fold

Lateral avulsion and phenolisation

Remove tourniquet and apply pressure to nail bed

Confirm haemostasis

Apply dressing

Patient given wound care and footwear advice

Aftercare

Following ingrown toenail surgery, appropriate advice on dressings and footwear should be given. Patients should be advised to re-attend if they develop increasing pain and signs of infection.

Hints and tips

- In chronic cases, lateral avulsion and phenolisation is recommended such that a 4 mm strip is cut from the lateral edge of the nail down to the germinal matrix; an incision must be made to the full length of the nail. A cotton bud soaked in phenol should be applied for 3 minutes to reach this germinal matrix. This helps achieve haemostasis as well as prevent re-growth.

- Excess phenol is deactivated by irrigation with an alcohol solution.

- The surrounding skin may be protected from tissue damage by the phenol using soft paraffin.

Shave excisions and curettage

Shave excisions

These may be carried out for skin tags with a narrow base. The skin lesions may or may not be anaesthetised. The skin tag is held with tissue forceps and the skin lesion is shaved or cut at the base using scissors or a scalpel blade. The blade is held horizontal to the skin surface. Direct pressure is usually adequate to control bleeding although electrocautery may be used. Alternatively, cautery excision may be employed.

A shave excision may also be used for benign skin lesions that are elevated, such as seborrhoeic keratoses. A surgical razor may also be used for this purpose. Generally, shave excisions are not carried out on naevi and care needs to be taken that the skin lesion undergoing a shave excision is benign. Although there is a risk of recurrence with shave excisions there is a minimal risk of scarring.

Punch biopsy

A punch biopsy where a core of tissue is excised may be used for diagnosis of a skin lesion or rash. Depending on the size of the punch biopsy, skin approximation with a simple interrupted suture may be required. This is generally carried out by a dermatologist.

Curettage

Curettage is less invasive when compared with excision and may be a good option for seborrhoeic keratoses and viral warts. Blood loss tends to be minimal and direct pressure, aluminium chloride or electrocautery may be used to aid haemostasis. As the dermis has not been breached, the cosmetic result is often better than with a more invasive approach.

It is possible to use curettage as a treatment for pyogenic granuloma. However, it should be remembered that a potential differential diagnosis of pyogenic granuloma may be an amelanotic melanoma and so I do not undertake surgical treatment for pyogenic granuloma. Furthermore, remember that 15% of cutaneous horns have histological changes of squamous cell carcinoma at the base, emphasising the need to send all specimens to histology.

It is recommended that keratoacanthomas are treated by excision even though there is usually a history of spontaneous regression. Excision is recommended because spontaneous regression may leave an unsightly scar and, moreover, these lesions may represent squamous cell carcinomas. However, in line with local guidance I do not undertake surgical treatment for keratoacanthomas but instead refer these cases to a dermatologist.

Cryotherapy

Cryotherapy usually involves the use of liquid nitrogen to freeze tissue, causing its destruction in a controlled way. Intra- and extracellular ice is created and the freezing and subsequent thawing of the tissue results in disruption of cell membranes. These processes create an inflammatory response.

Cryotherapy should only be used for lesions where a confident clinical diagnosis can be made. It may be used for benign skin lesions in primary care in certain patients because no histological diagnosis can be obtained. Because cryotherapy is painful, its use is best avoided in children.

An 'ice ball' or white ice field is maintained for the required length of time to create an inflammatory response. The length of time needed to destroy tissue relates to the lesion being treated. The freeze time is counted from when the skin lesion has turned white. Application may be by spray, probe or a cotton-tipped applicator, but the use of a cryospray is recommended because there is a greater level of control. Spray is directed from a distance of approximately 1 cm and because there is no direct patient contact, there is no risk of cross-contamination. Cryoprobes require longer freeze times and need to be autoclaved after use.

Following cryotherapy, patients should be advised that the thawing process may be painful and that signs of inflammation including blistering may develop within 2–3 hours; a patient information leaflet specific for cryo-therapy should be provided which outlines this. Patients should be advised to re-attend if they have particular concerns regarding healing.

Viral warts

Cryotherapy is often used in the treatment of viral warts. However, it should be remembered that most viral warts are self-limiting and treat-ment with salicylic acid preparations and duct tape are just as effective as cryotherapy.

Two freeze–thaw cycles are usually necessary, even for small viral warts. An 'ice ball' time of 5–10 seconds is usually sufficient for small viral warts, but up to 30 seconds is necessary for large plantar warts. In the case of genital warts, referral to a GUM clinic is recommended.

Solar and seborrhoeic keratoses

Solar keratoses are considered to be pre-malignant; however, the risk of progression to squamous cell carcinoma is unknown. They typically affect sun-exposed sites and may be textured, circumscribed and scaly. They are usually less than 1 cm in diameter. Solar keratoses may be treated with cryotherapy for up to 15 seconds; two freeze–thaw cycles may be required.

One cycle is usually sufficient for seborrhoeic keratoses, even if thick, but the 'ice ball' time is longer, at up to 25 seconds.

Other considerations

Verbal consent for cryotherapy is usually sufficient. Audit for cryotherapy should include freeze time, follow-up data and outcomes. Attention should be paid to health and safety guidance in relation to the storage and use of liquid nitrogen.

CHAPTER 3

Joint injections

General principles

Joint injections are commonly performed in general practice for a range of musculoskeletal problems and they form part of the minor surgery DES. A successful joint injection service relies on appropriate selection of patients following diagnosis. It is also dependent on the skill base of the clinician performing the procedure as well as their anatomical knowledge. Various courses are available for GPs to attend to learn about and practise joint injections[1] and practical experience may be gained while being overseen by a skilled clinician. Indications for joint injection include osteoarthritis, rheumatoid arthritis, synovitis, bursitis and tendinitis.

Joint injection may be therapeutic and joint aspiration may aid diagnosis. The commonest joint injections performed in general practice are those of the shoulder, knee and elbow. Obtaining a diagnosis involves history taking and a clinical examination that includes assessing active, passive and resisted movements at a joint. Diagnostic imaging may be helpful but is often unnecessary. A referral to secondary care should be considered if there is diagnostic doubt or if performing the required injection is outside the expertise of the clinician.

Remuneration for joint injections under the DES is in the order of £40 per joint injection and £40 per aspiration of bursa or effusion. Reimbursement can be obtained for the prescribing costs of the injections. Audit data should be collected regularly to assess outcome as well as possible complications. There is no specific accreditation process for performing joint injections, although local guidance advises that a sustained level of activity of at least 20 procedures per year, as well as evidence of relevant educational activities, should be carried out for continuing professional development. Local guidance may also be available to indicate which injections may be performed in general practice and when specialist referral may be more appropriate.

Evidence for joint injections

Evidence for the effectiveness of steroid joint injections is often anecdotal and there is little evidence comparing joint injection therapy with other interventions. The evidence that does exist suggests improvements in the

---

[1] Courses available through:

- the Royal College of General Practitioners: www.rcgp.org.uk/courses_events.aspx

- the British Institute of Musculoskeletal Medicine: www.bimm.org.uk/education

short term (Coombes *et al.*, 2010; Stephens *et al.*, 2008; Uthman *et al.*, 2003). The evidence for efficacy of intra-articular steroids in osteoarthritis is relatively weak (Creamer, 1997). However, according to Bellamy *et al.* (2005) the short-term benefit of intra-articular corticosteroids in treatment of knee osteoarthritis is well established. Stephens *et al.* (2008) report that corticosteroid injections are curative for de Quervain's tenosynovitis.

Effectiveness of joint injections is assessed by alleviation of pain and improving range of movement at a joint. The therapeutic response to corticosteroid injections is variable (Cardone and Tallia, 2002). Despite the lack of evidence for injection therapy it is widely practised. The variables in practice include choice of joint injection technique, volume and drug dosage to inject.

How often to inject

The recommended interval between intra-articular injections is 3 months, according Stephens *et al.* (2008). In my clinical practice, a large joint is injected no more than three times before referral to secondary care. Repeated joint injections should obviously not be carried out if there is no evidence of benefit. Injection frequency should take into consideration the underlying disease process and availability of other treatment options, as well as patient choice (Stephens *et al.*, 2008). Schumacher (2003) recommends that no more than three intra-articular steroid injections are performed in a year.

Contraindications

Absolute contraindications for joint injection include acute fracture, joint prosthesis and localised infection. Relative contraindications include poorly controlled diabetes, bleeding disorders, anticoagulation and joint osteoporosis. Systemic absorption of steroid following joint injection and joint damage should be considered when assessing patients who may be suitable for the procedure.

Risks and benefits of the procedure

The patient should undergo clinical assessment and if, after discussing possible management options, joint injection is being considered, the risks and benefits of the procedure should be discussed. Conservative measures such as maximal analgesia should ideally be trialled before proceeding to joint injection. Informed consent should be obtained, although this does not need to be in written form.

Risks of joint injection include:

- pain

- infection; joint sepsis is a rare complication

- steroid 'flare' after 24–36 hours; this is uncommon and thought to be a crystal-induced synovitis caused by preservatives in the injectable suspension (Genovese, 1998)

- neurovascular damage

- injury to cartilage

- tendon rupture and atrophy; injections into tendons should be avoided to reduce the risk of tendon rupture (Cardone and Tallia, 2002)

- lipodystrophy

- skin depigmentation; skin changes are more likely to occur in dark-skinned patients and where superficial areas are being injected, therefore it is preferable to use hydrocortisone in these cases.

Moreover, joint injection may not be effective in alleviating symptoms.

Systemic effects of steroid joint injection include vasovagal reaction, facial flushing and hypersensitivity reaction, with facial flushing being the commonest side-effect (Stephens *et al.*, 2008). Suppression of the hypothalamic–pituitary axis as a result of corticosteroid injection is unlikely to be of clinical significance. It is important to advise diabetic patients that glycaemic control may be affected following joint injection.

Steroid injections

The most commonly used steroids are hydrocortisone acetate 25 mg/ml (Hydrocortistab®), methylprednisolone 40 mg/ml (Depo-Medrone®) and triamcinolone acetonide at 10 mg/ml (Adcortyl®) and 40 mg/ml (Kenalog®). These agents vary in potency and solubility (see *Table 3.1*). Hydrocortisone is the least potent of these, followed by methylprednisolone, with triamcinolone being the most potent steroid that may be used. The less soluble the steroid used, the more likely it is that it will remain in the joint and so prolong the effect; triamcinolone is the least soluble of the commonly used

Table 3.1: **Commonly used steroids for injection therapy**

Steroid	Dose	
Hydrocortisone acetate 25 mg/ml (Hydrocortistab®)	10–25 mg for small joints	
	50 mg for large joints	Increasing potency
Methylprednisolone 40 mg/ml (Depo-Medrone®)	4–10 mg for small joints	Increasing duration of action
	20–80 mg for large joints	
Triamcinolone acetonide 10 mg/ml (Adcortyl®)	2.5–5 mg for small joints	Decreasing solubility
	5–15 mg for large joints	
Triamcinolone acetonide 40 mg/ml (Kenalog®)	5–10 mg for small joints	
	up to 40 mg for large joints	

injectable steroids (Stephens *et al.*, 2008). Low-solubility agents should not be used for soft tissue injection because there is an increased risk of surrounding tissue atrophy (Cardone and Tallia, 2002). Hydrocortisone has a short duration of action when compared to methylprednisolone and triamcinolone. The volume dose should also be considered when selecting an appropriate steroid for joint injection.

Soft tissue and small joint injections

For soft tissue and small joints, the following options may be considered:

- 10–25 mg hydrocortisone

- 4–10 mg methylprednisolone may be used for metacarpophalangeal and acromioclavicular joints

- 10–40 mg methylprednisolone may be used for the elbow and wrist

- 2.5–5 mg triamcinolone acetonide

Large joint injections

For large joints such as the knee and shoulder, the following options may be considered:

- 50 mg hydrocortisone

- 4–30 mg of methylprednisolone may be appropriate for intrabursal injection

- 20–80 mg of methylprednisolone

- 5–15 mg triamcinolone acetonide

In my clinical practice I usually use triamcinolone acetonide 40 mg/ml (Kenalog®) at entheses and small joints because injecting large volumes may cause pain and increase the risk of tendon rupture. For larger joints an increased volume can be helpful and this can be achieved by addition of local anaesthetic.

There is variation amongst clinicians as to which corticosteroid is favoured for injection as well as doses administered. Therefore any guidance given as to what may be administered should not be taken as absolute and clinical judgment should be exercised. Details of suggested needle length are given, but consideration should be given as to whether the needle chosen will be long enough to enter the joint, depending on body habitus.

It is common practice to mix local anaesthetic with corticosteroid for joint injections; this avoids injection of a highly concentrated suspension into a single area (Cardone and Tallia, 2002). Addition of local anaesthetic may also help differentiate between local and referred pain. Lidocaine (1 or 2%) is the most commonly used local anaesthetic because it has a rapid onset of action. Single dose ampoules are used both for local anaesthetic and steroid. Hydrocortisone and triamcinolone may be mixed with local anaes-thetic prior to administration, but methylprednisolone is not licensed for this. However, the manufacturer produces a ready-mixed preparation for the latter containing lidocaine (Depo-Medrone® with lidocaine).

Practical considerations

Joint injections should be performed using a sterile technique and sterile gloves. The steroid and local anaesthetic are drawn up with one needle and a new needle is then used to perform the injection. The point of insertion for joint injection may be marked by indentation or by a sterile marker pen. A 21-gauge needle (green in the UK) is often used to inject larger joints such as the knee and shoulder, and 23- or 25-gauge needles (blue and orange respectively in the UK) are usually more appropriate for smaller joints (Stephens et al., 2008). It is important that the needle is of sufficient length to reach the joint cavity; consideration should be given to this in patients with a raised BMI. An alcohol swab is commonly used to prepare the skin. Needle insertion is perpendicular to skin that is being stretched. Prior to injection, aspiration should be carried out to avoid inadvertent injection into a blood vessel.

Aftercare

When local anaesthesia is co-administered with corticosteroids, most patients experience rapid relief of symptoms due to the initial action of the local anaesthetic (Stephens *et al.*, 2008). Patients are advised that the local anaesthetic will wear off in a couple of hours. The effect of corticosteroid injection may become apparent after 48 hours but this is highly variable. A dressing is applied post-procedure and patients are advised to avoid strenuous activity for a few days and should be alerted to the signs of possible infection. Patients should be advised to report increased pain, fever and swelling after joint injection.

The line diagrams in the following chapter which show the sites of upper and lower limb joint injections do not always illustrate all muscles, to improve clarity for the reader.

CHAPTER 4

Steroid injections in the upper limb

Shoulder injection

Shoulder pain may be caused by a range of clinical problems: rotator cuff tendinitis, supraspinatus tendinitis causing impingement, bicipital tendinitis, frozen shoulder or adhesive capsulitis, subacromial bursitis and glenohumeral osteoarthritis, as well as osteoarthritis of the acromioclavicular joint. Neck examination should be performed as part of an assessment of the shoulder because referred pain is part of the differential diagnosis.

Shoulder joint injections should enter the joint capsule, but do not necessarily need to be in the glenohumeral joint space, which is narrow and may be difficult to access. Shoulder joint injections may be performed using the posterior, anterior or lateral approach. The posterior approach to the shoulder is the easiest injection technique because the joint space is wider.

Elbow, wrist and hand injection

Elbow injections may be used in the treatment of tennis elbow, golfer's elbow and olecranon bursitis. Wrist injections can be used in the treatment of carpal tunnel syndrome and De Quervain's tenosynovitis. Injections into the hand may be used to treat carpometacarpal joint osteoarthritis and trigger finger.

Posterior approach to shoulder

Technique

The patient is usually seated with the arm at their side and the shoulder externally rotated. The needle is inserted 2–3 cm below the posterolateral aspect of the acromion and medial to the head of the humerus (*Figs 4.1 and 4.2*). The needle is advanced in the direction of the coracoid process anteriorly.

Suggested doses

- Triamcinolone acetonide 40 mg with 4 ml of 1% lidocaine (total volume 5 ml), or

- Triamcinolone acetonide 10 mg/ml (in larger shoulders where more volume may be required) with 4 ml of 1% lidocaine (total volume 8 ml).

- Delivery: use 21G (green) needle, with a suggested needle length of 40 mm.

Aftercare

Stretching exercises, as pain allows.

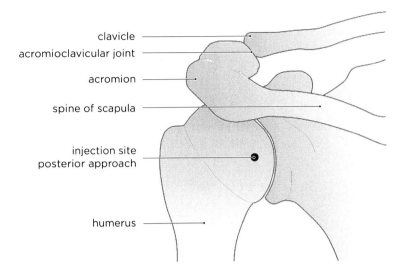

clavicle
acromioclavicular joint
acromion
spine of scapula
injection site
posterior approach
humerus

Figure 4.1: Posterior view of left shoulder.

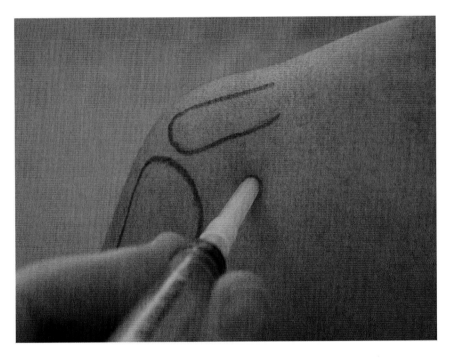

Figure 4.2: Photograph to demonstrate posterior approach for shoulder injection. Lines show acromion process and head of humerus.

Anterior approach to shoulder

Technique

The patient is usually seated with the arm at their side and the shoulder externally rotated. The needle is inserted below the acromion process, medial to the head of the humerus and 1 cm lateral to the coracoid process (*Figs 4.3* and *4.4*). The needle is advanced posteriorly at an angle that is slightly superior and lateral.

Suggested doses

- Triamcinolone acetonide 40 mg with 4 ml of 1% lidocaine (total volume 5 ml), or

- Triamcinolone acetonide 10 mg/ml (in larger shoulders where more volume may be required) with 4 ml of 1% lidocaine (total volume 8 ml)

- Delivery: use 21G (green) needle, with a suggested needle length of 40 mm.

Aftercare

Stretching exercises, as pain allows.

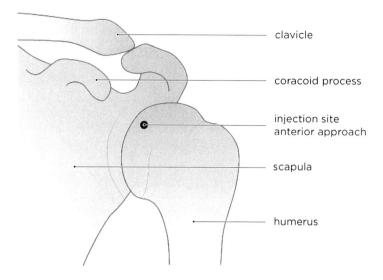

clavicle

coracoid process

injection site
anterior approach

scapula

humerus

Figure 4.3: Anterior view of the left shoulder.

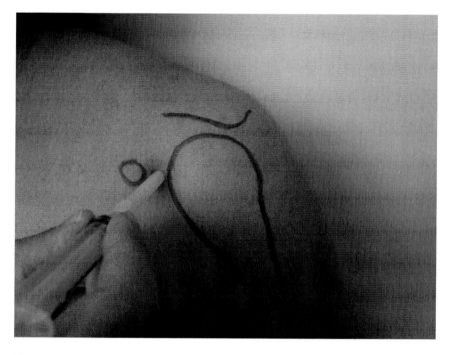

Figure 4.4: Anterior approach for shoulder injection. Lines show acromion
process, head of humerus and coracoid process.

Lateral or subacromial approach to shoulder

Subacromial injection may be helpful for rotator cuff pathology, calcific tendinitis, subacromial bursitis and adhesive capsulitis. Subacromial injection may be helpful in differentiating between shoulder weakness caused by impingement (where shoulder strength improves post-injection) and a true rotator cuff tear (where there is no improvement in strength post-injection).

Technique

The patient is seated with the arm at their side, not externally rotated. The needle is inserted in the horizontal plane below the acromion process in a slightly posterior direction along the line of the supraspinous fossa (*Figs 4.5* and *4.6*).

Suggested doses

- Triamcinolone acetonide 20 mg with 4.5 ml of 1% lidocaine (total volume 5 ml).

- Delivery: use 23G (blue) needle, with a suggested needle length of 30 mm.

Aftercare

It is advisable to avoid arm elevation above the shoulder for 2 weeks. Mobilisation exercises may be started, as pain allows.

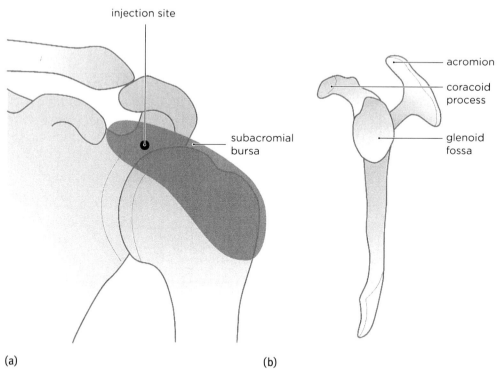

(a)   (b)

Figure 4.5: (a) Anterior view of left shoulder showing subacromial bursa, and (b) lateral view of the left shoulder.

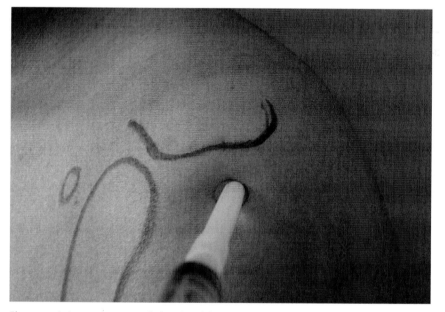

Figure 4.6: Lateral approach for shoulder injection. Lines show acromion process, head of humerus and coracoid process.

Acromioclavicular joint injection

Supraspinatus tendinitis may be demonstrated if the patient abducts their arm to 90° and pain is reproduced when resistance is applied. If pain is experienced from 90 to 180° this may be suggestive of acromioclavicular osteoarthritis. Furthermore, there is likely to be tenderness on palpation of the joint in acromioclavicular osteoarthritis.

Technique

The patient may be seated or supine for this joint injection; if the patient is seated with their affected arm hanging down, this opens up the joint space. The joint space should be palpated and the needle advanced either from an anterior or superior position (*Figs 4.7* and *4.8*). Acromioclavicular joint injection may be difficult if there is obstruction by an osteophyte.

Suggested doses

A small volume is used to inject the acromioclavicular joint because the space is small when compared to that of the shoulder.

- Triamcinolone acetonide 10 mg with 0.75 ml 2% lidocaine (total volume 1 ml).

- Delivery: use 25G (orange) needle, with a suggested needle length of 16 mm.

Aftercare

The affected shoulder may be rested for a week before gentle mobilisation of the joint.

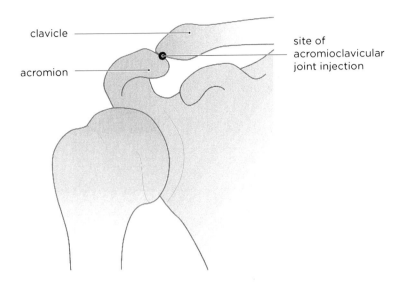

clavicle

acromion

site of
acromioclavicular
joint injection

Figure 4.7: Anterior view of right shoulder with acromioclavicular joint injection site shown.

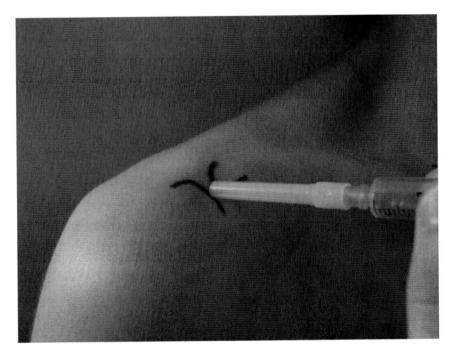

Figure 4.8: Acromioclavicular joint injection.

Injection for bicipital tendinitis

If shoulder pain is experienced on forearm flexion and supination with the elbow bent at 90° against resistance, this is suggestive of bicipital tendinitis or inflammation of the long head of the biceps muscle. Moreover, there will be tenderness on palpation between the greater and lesser tubercles of the head of the humerus, i.e. overlying the bicipital groove.

Technique

The arm is externally rotated and the bicipital groove palpated, the needle is inserted at the point of maximal tenderness and directed upwards at 30°. The area in and around the bicipital groove is infiltrated (*Figs 4.9* and *4.10*). Injecting under resistance should be avoided to reduce the risk of tendon rupture.

Suggested doses

- Triamcinolone acetonide 10 mg with 0.75 ml of 2% lidocaine (total volume 1 ml).

- Delivery: use 23G (blue) needle, with suggested needle length of 25 mm.

Aftercare

Relative rest is advised for a week followed by a return to usual activity.

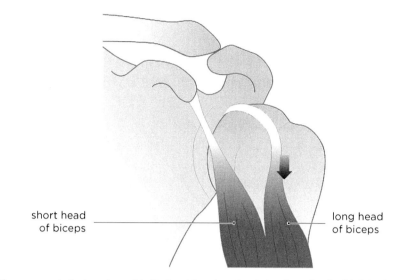

short head
of biceps

long head
of biceps

Figure 4.9: Anterior view of left shoulder showing injection site for bicipital tendinitis, between the greater and lesser tuberosities of the humerus.

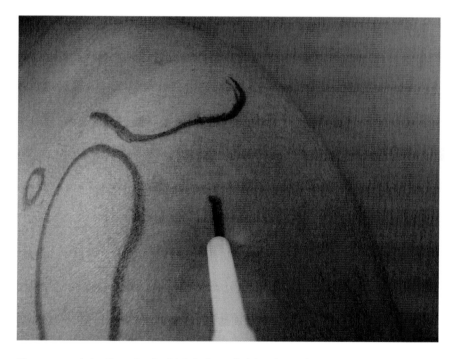

Figure 4.10: Injection site for bicipital tendinitis. Lines show acromion process, head of humerus, coracoid process and bicipital groove.

Injection for tennis elbow (lateral epicondylitis)

Pain is localised to the lateral epicondyle of the humerus in tennis elbow.

Technique

The patient may be seated or supine with the elbow flexed to 45° and the wrist pronated. The needle is inserted at the lateral epicondyle at the point of maximal tenderness on palpation, until the level of the periosteum (*Figs 4.11* and *4.12*). The needle is fanned subcutaneously at other points of tenderness, i.e. without the need to re-insert the needle. Local anaesthesia may be infiltrated initially in areas of tenderness, followed by steroid injection, or they may be co-administered. Lipodystrophy may be caused if there is inadvertent subcutaneous injection of steroid.

Suggested doses

- Triamcinolone acetonide 10 mg with 0.75 ml of 2% lidocaine (total volume 1 ml).

- Delivery: use 25G (orange) needle, with a suggested needle length of 16 mm.

Aftercare

Relative rest is advised for 1–2 weeks, and the activity which caused the tendinopathy should be avoided. Lifting is performed with the palm facing upwards so that the flexor muscles are used instead of the extensors.

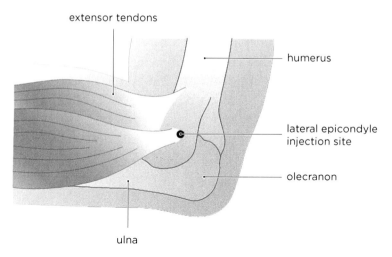

extensor tendons

humerus

lateral epicondyle
injection site

olecranon

ulna

Figure 4.11: Lateral view of the left elbow showing the injection site for lateral epicondylitis.

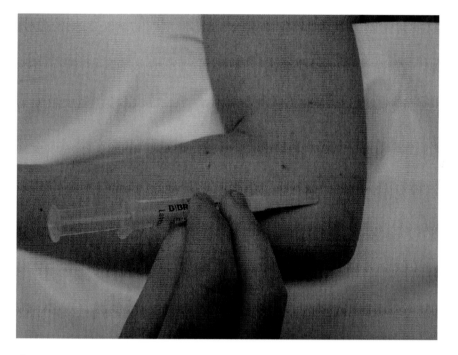

Figure 4.12: Injection site for tennis elbow at lateral epicondyle.

Injection for golfer's elbow (medial epicondylitis)

Pain is localised to the medial epicondyle of the humerus in golfer's elbow.

Technique

The patient may be seated or supine. The arm should be abducted, the elbow flexed to 45° and the hand supinated. The needle is inserted at the medial epicondyle at the point of maximal tenderness on palpation, until the level of the periosteum (*Figs 4.13* and *4.14*). The needle is fanned subcutaneously at other points of tenderness, taking care to avoid the ulnar nerve which is posterior to the medial epicondyle. If there is inadvertent contact with the ulnar nerve, the patient will complain of paraesthesia and the needle should be repositioned.

Suggested doses

- Triamcinolone acetonide 10 mg with 0.75 ml of 2% lidocaine (total volume 1 ml).

- Delivery: use 25G (orange) needle, with a suggested needle length of 16 mm.

Aftercare

Relative rest is advised for 1–2 weeks, followed by stretching and strengthening exercises.

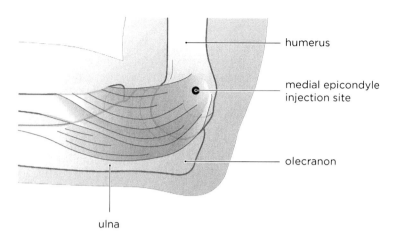

humerus

medial epicondyle
injection site

olecranon

ulna

Figure 4.13: Medial view of right elbow showing injection site for medial
epicondylitis.

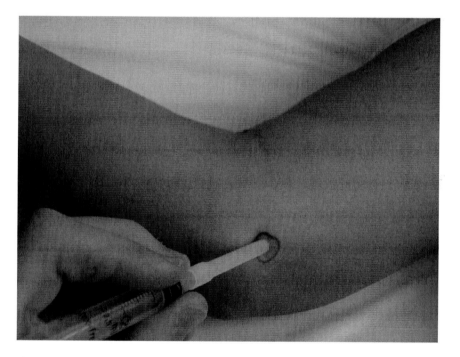

Figure 4.14: Injection site for golfer's elbow at medial epicondyle.

Injection for olecranon bursitis

The olecranon bursa is superficial to the olecranon process and extra-articular to the elbow joint. A needle may easily be inserted into the olecranon bursa if aspiration is required to relieve pain and swelling. Steroid injection may also be helpful.

Technique

The injection is performed with the arm flexed as much as possible (*Figs 4.15* and *4.16*). The needle is inserted at the point of maximal fluctuance. A pressure dressing is applied post-procedure.

Suggested doses

- Triamcinolone acetonide 20 mg with 1.5 ml of 2% lidocaine (total volume 2 ml).

- Delivery: use 23G (blue) needle, with a suggested needle length of 25 mm.

Aftercare

Relative rest is advised for a week, followed by a return to usual activity. Leaning on the affected elbow should initially be avoided.

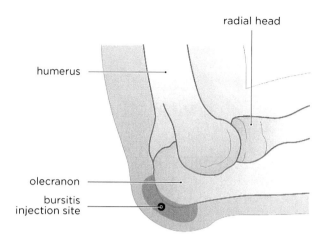

Figure 4.15: Lateral view of right elbow showing injection site for olecranon bursitis.

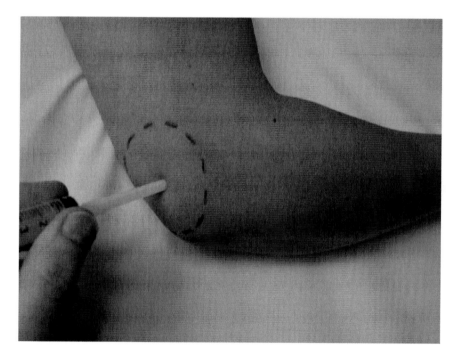

Figure 4.16: Injection site for olecranon bursitis.

Injection for carpal tunnel syndrome

Steroid injection is performed with the palm facing upwards. Local anaesthesia is not generally used because, in this case, it will exacerbate symptoms of carpal tunnel syndrome. It should be noted that inadvertent steroid injection into the median nerve may cause a chronic paraesthesia and therefore only experienced clinicians should attempt steroid injections to alleviate carpal tunnel syndrome.

Technique

The wrist is dorsiflexed to 30°. The needle is inserted at 30° on the ulnar side of the palmaris longus tendon at the proximal wrist crease (*Figs 4.17* and *4.18*). It is aimed towards the tip of the ring finger. In the absence of the palmaris longus tendon, the needle is inserted on the ulnar side of the midline of the wrist. The median nerve lies posterior to the palmaris longus tendon at the wrist in up to 90% of patients; if there is pain or paraesthesia on needle insertion this suggests contact with the median nerve and so the needle should be withdrawn and re-inserted. To avoid inadvertent injection into a tendon, the injection should not be given against resistance.

Suggested doses

- Triamcinolone acetonide 20 mg (total volume 0.5 ml).

- Delivery: use 23G (blue) needle, with a suggested needle length of 30 mm.

Aftercare

Rest is advised for one week, followed by a return to usual activity.

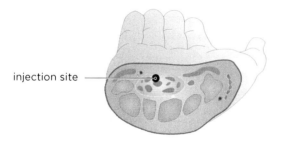

injection site

Figure 4.17: Injection site for carpal tunnel syndrome in right hand.

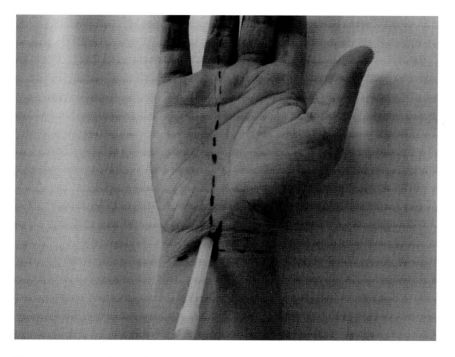

Figure 4.18: Carpal tunnel syndrome injection site. Lines show palmaris longus tendon, proximal wrist crease and line towards ring finger.

Injection for De Quervain's tenosynovitis

De Quervain's tenosynovitis affects the abductor pollicis longus and extensor pollicis brevis tendons where the radial styloid is traversed. Pain is reproduced when the patient makes a fist with the thumb in their palm and ulnar-deviates their flexed wrist.

Technique

The needle is inserted proximal to the first metacarpal on the extensor surface at 30°, along the line of the tendon distal to the point of maximal tenderness (*Figs 4.19* and *4.20*). The injection is administered in the tendon sheath. The effect of injecting steroid into the sheath should become apparent visually as a bulge is produced. Care should be taken to avoid inadvertent injection into the tendon itself, and the risk of this is minimised by avoiding injecting against resistance.

Suggested doses

- Triamcinolone acetonide 10 mg with 0.75 ml of 2% lidocaine (total volume 1 ml).

- Delivery: use 25G (orange) needle, with a suggested needle length of 16 mm.

Aftercare

The hand should be rested for one week and the activity that triggered the tenosynovitis avoided. Strengthening exercises may be helpful thereafter.

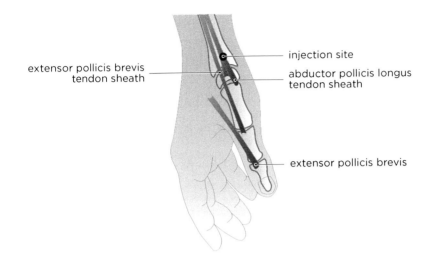

extensor pollicis brevis
tendon sheath

injection site

abductor pollicis longus
tendon sheath

extensor pollicis brevis

Figure 4.19: Injection site for De Quervain's tenosynovitis.

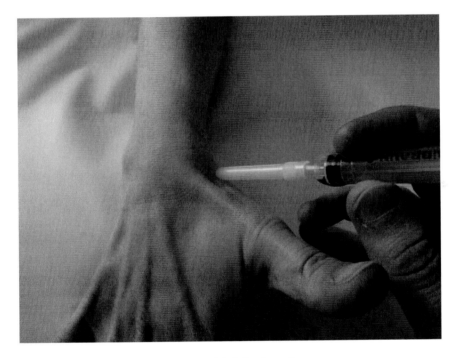

Figure 4.20: De Quervain's tenosynovitis injection site.

Injection for first carpometacarpal joint osteoarthritis

Osteoarthritis of the first carpometacarpal joint presents with localised tenderness on thumb abduction and extension.

Technique

The thumb should be tucked into the palm; the joint line on the lateral aspect of the thumb is palpated (*Figs 4.21* and *4.22*). Traction can be applied to the thumb to further open the joint space. The abductor pollicis tendon is identified to avoid inadvertent injection into this. The joint space is small so only a small volume of steroid is injected.

Interphalangeal joint injection may be considered for rheumatoid arthritis affecting the small joints of the hand.

Suggested doses

- Triamcinolone acetonide 10 mg with 0.75 ml of 2% lidocaine (total volume 1 ml).

- Delivery: use 25G (orange) needle, with a suggested needle length of 16 mm.

Aftercare

The thumb is taped using a spica technique for a few days in order to support the proximal metacarpophalangeal joint of the thumb. Gentle mobilisation is then advised.

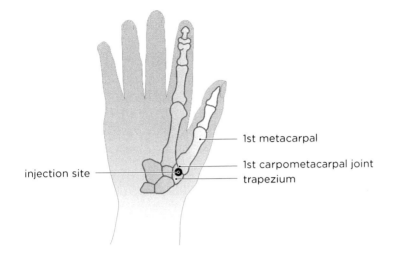

1st metacarpal

1st carpometacarpal joint

injection site

trapezium

Figure 4.21: Injection site for first carpometacarpal joint injection.

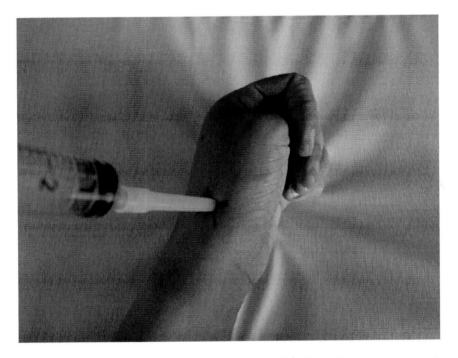

Figure 4.22: First carpometacarpal joint injection site. Lines show trapezium and base of first metacarpal.

Injection for trigger finger

Trigger finger is a tenosynovitis that may affect any of the flexor tendons.

Technique

The needle is inserted in the crease overlying the metacarpophalangeal joint and advanced proximally (*Figs 4.23* and *4.24*); this is particularly straightforward if a nodule can be felt in the palm of the hand because the needle can simply be advanced in the direction of this. Care must be taken to avoid inadvertent steroid injection into the tendon.

Suggested doses

- Triamcinolone acetonide 10 mg with 0.25 ml of 2% lidocaine (total volume 0.5 ml).

- Delivery: use 25G (orange) needle, with a suggested needle length of 16 mm.

Aftercare

Relative rest for a few days is advised and then usual activity may be resumed.

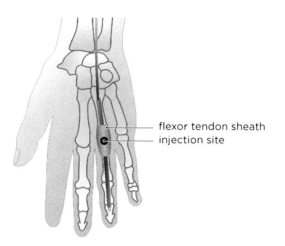

flexor tendon sheath
injection site

Figure 4.23: Injection site for trigger finger in the right hand.

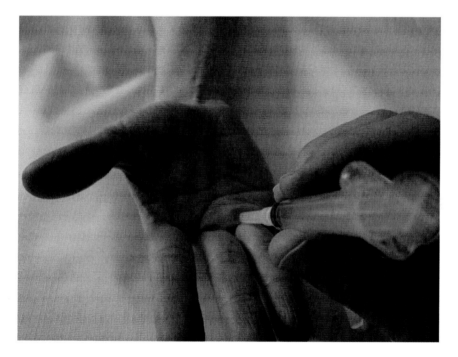

Figure 4.24: Trigger finger injection site.

CHAPTER 5

Steroid injections in the lower limb

Featured approaches

Injection for trochanteric bursitis

Trochanteric bursitis may be suspected if lateral hip pain is localised to the greater trochanter. The bursa may be detected by fluctuance on palpation, and a clear yellow fluid is often found on aspiration.

Technique

The patient is placed in the lateral recumbent position with the hip flexed to 30–50° and the knee flexed to 60–90°. The needle is inserted perpendicular to the skin at the point of maximal tenderness overlying the greater trochanter (*Figs 5.1* and *5.2*). The needle is inserted until bone is reached; on slight withdrawal of the needle fluid should be aspirated before the injection is given, using a new syringe but the same needle. The injection is done by feeling for an area of no resistance.

Suggested doses

- Triamcinolone acetonide 20 mg with 1.5 ml of 2% lidocaine (total volume 2 ml).

- Delivery: use 23G (blue) needle, with a suggested needle length of 30 mm.

Aftercare

Relative rest for one week is advised and then usual activities may be resumed.

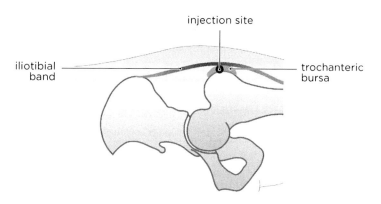

injection site

iliotibial band

trochanteric bursa

Figure 5.1: Injection site for trochanteric bursitis.

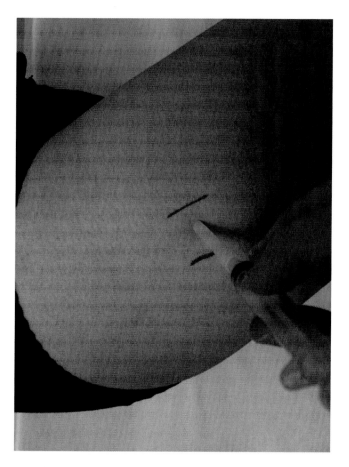

Figure 5.2: Trochanteric bursitis injection site in right hip with patient in lateral position.

Injection for meralgia paraesthetica

Meralgia paraesthetica is a painful mononeuropathy of the lateral cutaneous nerve of the thigh, caused by its compression as it passes under or through the inguinal ligament. Management of the condition may include weight loss and oral analgesia. However, in the case of more severe symptoms a nerve block may be helpful in providing temporary relief.

Technique

An area of tenderness is identified 10 cm below and medial to the anterior superior iliac spine and infiltrated with steroid with the patient supine (*Figs 5.3* and *5.4*). Injection is around the lateral cutaneous nerve of the thigh and care must be taken to avoid inadvertent injection into the nerve.

Suggested doses

- Triamcinolone acetonide 20 mg (total volume 0.5 ml).

- Delivery: use 21G (green) needle, with a suggested needle length of 50 mm.

Aftercare

Weight loss and avoidance of tightly fitted clothing may be helpful.

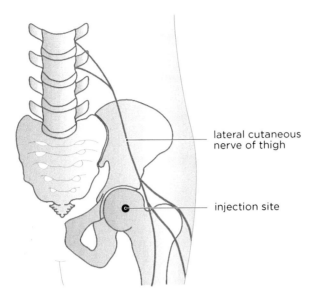

Figure 5.3: Injection site for meralgia paraesthetica.

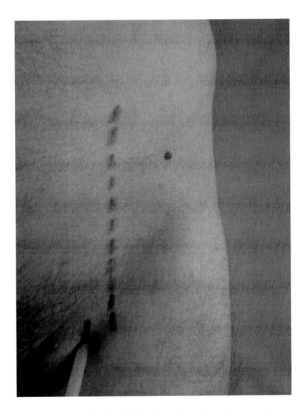

Figure 5.4: Meralgia paraesthetica injection site. Line shows site 10 cm below and medial to the anterior superior iliac spine.

Injection for iliotibial band syndrome

Inflammation of the distal portion of the iliotibial tendon as it rubs against the lateral femoral condyle may cause iliotibial band syndrome, which is an overuse phenomenon that occurs due to repetitive extension and flexion of the knee. It may be seen in long-distance runners and cyclists. The bursa is close to the iliotibial band above the lateral condyle of the femur.

Technique

The injection may be done with the patient in the supine position with the knee in a slightly flexed position with a pillow or rolled towel in the popliteal space. The needle is inserted into the bursa by traversing the tendon to reach bone on the lateral side of the femur (*Figs 5.5* and *5.6*).

Suggested doses

- Triamcinolone acetonide 20 mg and 1.5 ml 2% lidocaine (total volume 2 ml).

- Delivery: use 23G (blue) needle, with a suggested needle length of 25 mm.

Aftercare

The patient is advised to rest for 1–2 weeks, and this is then followed by stretching and strengthening exercises.

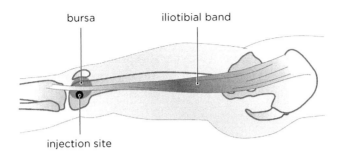

Figure 5.5: Lateral view of injection site for iliotibial band syndrome.

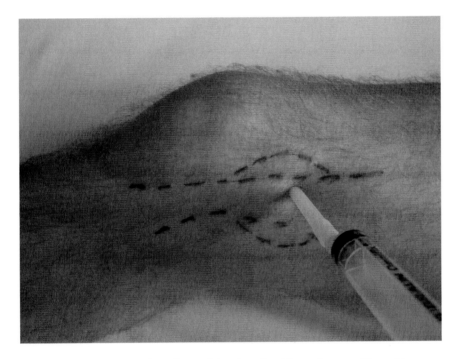

Figure 5.6: Iliotibial band syndrome injection site. Lines show position of bursa and iliotibial band.

Injection for the knee joint

Knee joint aspiration may be therapeutic in the case of a tense effusion causing pain, and an aspirate sent to the laboratory for analysis may be diagnostic.

Technique

Aspiration and injection may be done with the patient in the supine position with the knee in a slightly flexed position with a pillow or rolled towel in the popliteal space. The margin of the patella is palpated and the needle is inserted below its superior border (*Figs 5.7* and *5.8*). The needle may be inserted from the lateral or the medial side, and the needle is advanced in the horizontal plane behind the patella.

Dependent on the size of effusion to be drained, a 3-way connector between needle and syringe may be helpful. In the absence of this a further syringe may be connected to the needle to continue to drain a large effusion.

Suggested doses

- Triamcinolone acetonide 40 mg (as Adcortyl®) and 6 ml of 1% lidocaine; total volume: 10 ml; an increased volume is required for knee joint injection due to a large synovial surface area.

- Delivery: use 21G (green) needle, with a suggested needle length of 40 mm.

Aftercare

Avoidance of excessive weight-bearing activity for one week, followed by mobilisation.

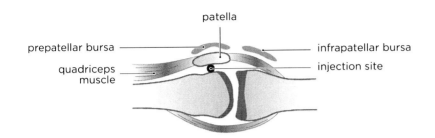

prepatellar bursa — infrapatellar bursa

patella

quadriceps — injection site
muscle

Figure 5.7: Aspiration and injection site for the knee – medial approach.

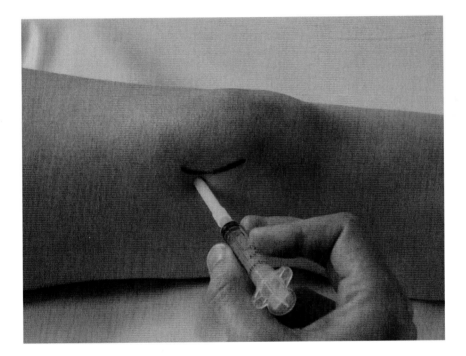

Figure 5.8: Knee injection and aspiration site from the medial side.

Injection for the ankle joint

Ankle joint injections may be helpful for rheumatoid arthritis or osteoarthritis. Arthropathies affecting the ankle joint usually respond well to joint injection. However, the ankle is prone to infection and so a strict aseptic technique is required. It is advisable to refer ankle joint injections to secondary care.

Technique

The patient is supine with the knee flexed. The needle is inserted in the joint space between the tibia and talus using an anterior approach. The needle is placed between the tibialis anterior and extensor hallucis longus tendons (*Figs 5.9* and *5.10*).

Suggested doses

- Triamcinolone acetonide 30 mg and 1.75 ml 2% lidocaine (total volume 2.5 ml).

- Delivery: use 23G (blue) needle, with a suggested needle length of 30 mm.

Aftercare

The patient is advised to avoid excessive weight-bearing exercise for one week.

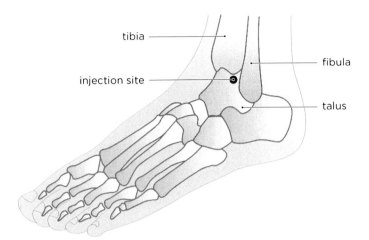

tibia

fibula

injection site

talus

Figure 5.9: Injection site for the left ankle joint.

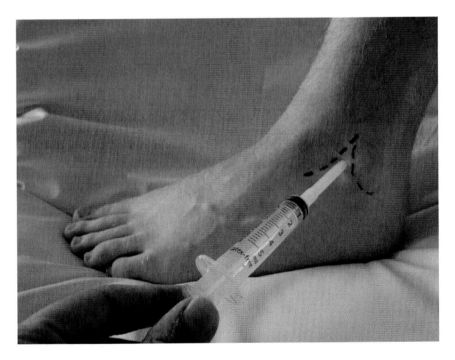

Figure 5.10: Left ankle joint injection site showing an anterior approach. Lines show tibia and fibula just above talus.

Injection for posterior tibial tendinitis

Posterior tibial tendinitis is a tenosynovitis affecting the foot and ankle. It may be caused by an acute injury or through overuse in patients who undertake high impact sports. Pain is localised along the course of the posterior tibial tendon along the back and inside of the foot and ankle. The injection for this is in the tendon sheath space. The needle is inserted below the medial malleolus in line with the posterior tibial tendon in a proximal direction. This injection is not often performed in general practice.

Injection for tarsal tunnel syndrome

Tarsal tunnel syndrome is a compression neuropathy of the tibial nerve or its branches as it traverses the flexor retinaculum at the level of the ankle or more distally. The flexor retinaculum forms the roof of the tarsal tunnel and it consists of the deep fascia of the leg and ankle. Tarsal tunnel syndrome may be caused by osteoarthritis, post-traumatic ankle injuries or tenosynovitis.

Compressive symptoms include numbness and pain, usually along the medial border of the foot. This condition is analogous to carpal tunnel syndrome of the wrist.

Steroid injection may be helpful, but care must be taken to avoid inadvertent nerve injury during injection. This is an uncommon compression neuropathy and injection therapy is not often performed. If conservative measures are unsuccessful, referral for tarsal tunnel release should be considered.

Injection for plantar fasciitis

Steroid injection may be helpful for plantar fasciitis. However, it is particularly painful for the patient and is best avoided in general practice.

CHAPTER 6

Long-acting reversible methods of contraception

Long-acting reversible contraception (LARC) methods include the intra-muscular injection of medroxyprogesterone (Depo-Provera), the intra-uterine device/system, and the subdermal contraceptive implant. Provision of the latter two services is beyond that of standard core services because enhanced skills and training are required for delivery. Contraceptive service providers who do not provide LARC methods within their own practice or service should have an agreed mechanism in place for referring women on.

Provision of LARC methods in general practice often forms part of a Local Enhanced Service (LES). The NICE LARC methods guideline (NICE, 2006, CG30: *Long-acting reversible contraception*) states that increasing the uptake of LARC methods will reduce the numbers of unintended pregnancies. All currently available LARC methods are more cost-effective than the combined oral contraceptive pill at 1 year of use. Moreover, intrauterine devices, the intrauterine system and implants are more cost-effective than injectable contraceptives.

As part of the service there should be a system for keeping records of patient assessment and follow-up, or recall arrangements. In addition to provision of advanced family planning, all patients treated should undergo a sexual history review and be offered opportunistic screening for sexually transmitted infections.

Pre-requisites

An appropriate room fitted with a couch, as well as the special equipment required for intrauterine device or implant fitting or removal, is required for this LES. Special equipment includes vaginal specula, cervical dilators and resuscitation equipment. An appropriately trained nurse may be present to support the patient and assist the clinician during the procedure; note that there is no specific guidance regarding the assistant's role for these procedures except that they should be familiar with procedures and what is required for them.

In order to deliver the service, the clinician must have relevant accreditation, i.e. hold the Diploma of the Faculty of Sexual and Reproductive Healthcare (DFSRH). The training for this involves e-learning for theoretical background knowledge and small group workshops, in addition to clinical experience and assessment. Further details are available on the Faculty of Sexual and Reproductive Healthcare of the Royal College of Obstetricians and Gynaecologists website (www.fsrh.org). Furthermore, a Letter of Competence (LoC) in the required procedure is needed from the FSRH.

Subdermal contraceptive implant techniques

Requirements for gaining the LoC in subdermal contraceptive implant techniques include self-directed theoretical training and model arm training, and at least two consecutive insertion procedures must be observed by an approved trainer. Furthermore, two consecutive removal procedures must also be observed by an approved trainer. Re-certification involves ongoing continuing professional development as well as production of a log of clinical experience; a log covering a consecutive 12 month period will need to show a minimum of six procedures, including at least one insertion and one removal.

Intrauterine techniques

Requirements for gaining the LoC in intrauterine techniques involve theoretical training, model uterus training, and a minimum of seven competent insertions of intrauterine devices in conscious women observed by an approved trainer. The observed insertions must include at least two different currently available devices. Moreover, insertion of hormonal and copper devices should be observed. Re-certification for this LoC also involves ongoing continuing professional development in addition to the production of a log of clinical experience; a log covering a consecutive 12 month period will need to show a minimum of 12 insertions of at least two different types of device.

Local guidance from the Primary Care Organisation for the running of a sexual health or LARC enhanced service should be consulted. In addition, local guidance should be referred to with regard to remuneration as this may vary, but is typically:

- insertion of an intrauterine device: £100–130
- insertion of a subdermal implant: £40–50
- removal of a subdermal implant: £60–80.

Subdermal contraceptive implant (Nexplanon®)

Nexplanon® is a progestogen-only implant whose contraceptive effect is primarily achieved by inhibition of ovulation. It is preloaded in a sterile disposable applicator to facilitate subdermal insertion and is radio-opaque, unlike its predecessor Implanon. The implant is 4 cm long and 2 mm in diameter and contains 68 mg of etonogestrel. It is licensed as a method of contraception for up to 3 years. It is placed subdermally at the inner aspect of the upper arm to avoid neurovascular structures between the biceps and triceps muscle. This subdermal placement also reduces the risk of implant migration. Further information on the Nexplanon® implant is available on eMC[1].

The timing and appropriateness of insertion is dependent on the patient's contraceptive and medical history; for example, if a woman has not used hormonal contraception in the last month, the implant should be inserted between days 1 and 5 of the menstrual cycle. It is usual to offer patients pre-procedure implant counselling to discuss methods of contraception that are appropriate for their requirements, so that the risks and benefits of each method can be discussed fully. In a clinically appropriate situation following pre-procedure counselling, a consent form should be completed (see *Appendix 3: Consent to insertion of contraceptive implant form*).

Nexplanon® insertion

Nexplanon® insertion is performed under aseptic conditions with the preloaded applicator; it is recommended that the procedure is performed by the operator in a seated position. The patient lies on her back on the examination couch with the non-dominant arm flexed at the elbow and externally rotated so that her hand is positioned next to her head. At the inner aspect of the non-dominant upper arm about 8–10 cm proximal to the medial epicondyle of the humerus, the insertion site is marked (*Fig. 6.1*). A second site may be marked to help guide direction of insertion. The area is cleaned with an antiseptic and local anaesthetic given. The transparent cap is removed from the needle which contains the implant (*Fig. 6.2*).

The skin around the insertion site is stretched and the needle inserted at about 30°. When the needle is positioned subdermally, the applicator should be lowered to a horizontal position. The needle is inserted to its full length subdermally. At this point the slider at the top of the applicator should be unlocked by slightly depressing it (*Fig. 6.3*).

This is then retracted fully, thereby leaving the implant in its final position and the needle inside the body of the applicator. Prior to dressings being applied, the presence of the implant should be confirmed by palpation after

---

[1] Full details on the Nexplanon® implant can be found at: www.medicines.org.uk/EMC/medicine/23824/SPC/ Nexplanon®+68+mg+implant+for+subdermal+use [last updated 23/10/2012; last accessed 9/1/2013].

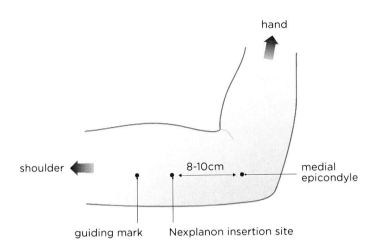

Figure 6.1: Nexplanon® insertion site at inner aspect of non-dominant upper arm.

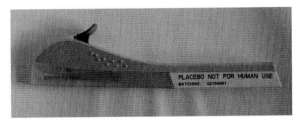

Figure 6.2: Implant insertion device with transparent cap *in situ* shielding needle.

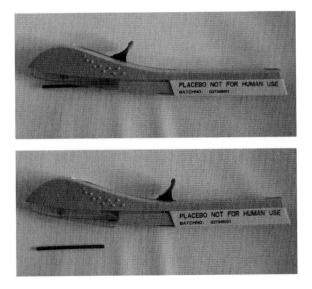

Figure 6.3: The needle retracts when the slider is partially depressed (top) and when the slider is moved fully back the implant is left *in situ* and the needle retracts inside the applicator (bottom).

insertion; the patient should also be encouraged to check that they can palpate the implant *in situ* post-procedure.

Nexplanon® removal

The location of the implant should always be known prior to removal and, for removal in general practice, the implant must be palpable subdermally.

Prior to removal, the site is cleaned with antiseptic; the distal end of the implant is marked with a sterile marker. Local anaesthetic is given where the incision will be made and underneath the implant, to keep it close to the skin surface. A small incision is made at the distal end with a scalpel whilst pushing down at the proximal end of the implant. The tip is grasped using forceps and removed. The implant may need to be freed by tissue dissection if it has become encapsulated; usually this is related to the length of time the implant has been *in situ*. After removal, dressings are applied. A new implant may be inserted immediately after the old implant is removed using the same incision if appropriate.

Intrauterine system (Mirena®)

The levonorgestrel intrauterine system (IUS) or Mirena® coil may be used for contraception, primary menorrhagia and endometrial protection during oestrogen replacement therapy. The IUS prevents endometrial proliferation, thickens cervical mucus and may suppress ovulation. It is effective for 5 years when indicated for contraception and primary menorrhagia and for 4 years if being used for endometrial protection during oestrogen replacement therapy. The timing and appropriateness of insertion should be evaluated pre-procedure with counselling to ensure suitability for this LARC method. Furthermore, the risks and benefits of this procedure should be discussed. Further information on the Mirena® coil is available on eMC[2].

The risks of Mirena® insertion include: pain, bleeding, uterine perforation, vasovagal reaction, pelvic infection, expulsion, lost threads, hormonal side-effects, ovarian cysts and contraceptive failure. Written consent for the procedure should be obtained from appropriately prepared patients. A risk assessment and screening for sexually transmitted infections are carried out.

---

[2] Full details on the Mirena® can be found at: www.medicines.org.uk/EMC/medicine/1829/SPC/Mirena [last updated 16/7/2012; last accessed 9/1/2013].

Mirena® coil insertion

The patient should undergo bimanual examination to assess the size and position of the uterus. The cervix is visualised using a speculum, then the cervix and vagina are cleaned with an antiseptic solution. The uterus is stabilised by holding the anterior lip of the cervix with a tenaculum or other forceps. Gentle counter traction on the cervix is required during Mirena® coil insertion. The depth and direction of the uterine cavity is assessed by passing a uterine sound through the cervical canal to the uterine fundus; cervical dilatation may be necessary with or without paracervical block. This will also allow detection of intrauterine abnormalities.

Mirena® coil insertion is undertaken using a sterile technique. The product consists of an IUS loaded at the tip of the inserter (*Fig. 6.4*). The inserter comprises an insertion tube with plunger and scale, flange, body and slider. The IUS system has a hormone–elastomer core mounted on a T-body. The T-body has a loop at one end where the removal threads are attached and two arms at the other end.

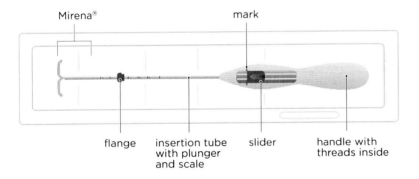

Figure 6.4: Mirena® insertion pack.

The slider is pushed forward to load the Mirena® into the insertion tube; whilst holding the slider in position, the upper edge of the flange is set to the uterine depth. Whilst continuing to hold the slider in position, the inserter is passed through the cervix until the flange is approximately 2 cm from the uterine cervix. The slider is pulled to the mark to allow the horizontal arms of the Mirena® to open whilst maintaining the position of the inserter. At this point the inserter is carefully advanced towards the uterine fundus until the flange is touching the cervix. The Mirena® can then be released by pulling the slider all the way down; with the slider in this position the inserter is removed (*Fig. 6.5*). The threads are cut to leave approximately 2 cm outside the cervix.

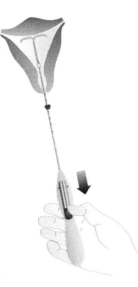

Figure 6.5: Inserter being held in place and the Mirena® being released by pulling back on the slider.

Mirena® coil removal

The Mirena® is removed by applying gentle traction on the threads with forceps. After removal, the IUS should be inspected to check that it has been fully removed.

Intrauterine devices

Intrauterine devices (IUDs) refer to copper-containing devices which can be used for emergency contraception and non-hormonal contraception. There are several copper-containing devices available and the choice of which to use may be determined by uterine length. It is thought that copper ions interfere with sperm motility and cause a foreign body type reaction. IUDs are inserted into the uterus using a technique for insertion that is similar to that required for the IUS; however, individual protocols should still be consulted.

CHAPTER 7

Other procedures

Nasal cautery

Nasal cautery to Little's area may be used to prevent recurrent bleeding from a small blood vessel. This procedure takes a few minutes and may be carried out in general practice.

An appropriate light source and a nasal speculum are used to look for an obvious bleeding point. This technique should not be used if there is active bleeding. If nasal cautery is appropriate, the area should be anaesthetised first: cotton wool impregnated with local anaesthetic may be packed into the nostril or, alternatively, the area may be sprayed with lidocaine and phenylephrine. Once anaesthetised, cautery can be carried out, either chemically with a silver nitrate stick, or an electrocautery needle may be gently applied to the bleeding point. The upper lip may be protected from chemical burns by applying petroleum jelly. It is not advisable to perform nasal cautery on both sides of the nasal septum at the same time. Post-procedure application of topical antibiotic such as Naseptin® (which contains chlorhexidine and neomycin) is generally recommended. Complications of nasal cautery include symptom recurrence and so re-cauterisation may be necessary. Repeat procedures may increase the risk of septal perforation.

Granuloma tissue may be cauterised in a similar manner.

Microsuction of the external auditory canal

Microsuction of the external auditory canal for removal of ear wax and debris in the case of otitis externa may also be carried out in general practice if the clinician has the appropriate skills required to do so.

Carpal tunnel decompression

Carpal tunnel syndrome may be characterised by pain, paraesthesia and weakness in the median nerve distribution of the hand. It is one of the most common entrapment neuropathies. The clinical diagnosis may be supported by provocative tests such as Phalen's test, Tinel's test and the carpal compression test, as well as nerve conduction studies.

It may be managed conservatively by wrist splinting and/or steroid injection, dependent on clinical context and severity of symptoms. For example, carpal tunnel syndrome in pregnancy is likely to be transient and so conservative management may be the most appropriate option.

It should be noted that inadvertent steroid injection into the median nerve may cause a chronic paraesthesia and therefore only experienced clinicians should attempt steroid injections to alleviate carpal tunnel syndrome.

Surgery is recommended if there is evidence of median nerve denervation. Carpal tunnel decompression may be performed using an open or endoscopic technique to divide the flexor retinaculum, but in general practice only open carpal tunnel decompression is an option. Whilst recovery time may be faster for endoscopic decompression, it has a higher complication rate. Risks include recurrent symptoms, acute and/or chronic pain, infection and bleeding, as well as nerve and tendon damage.

The procedure

The procedure may be carried out under local anaesthesia; this may be infiltrated into the carpal tunnel as well as injected subcutaneously. Local anaesthesia may be used with or without a tourniquet.

A longitudinal incision is made in the base of the palm in line with the flexed ring finger up until the distal wrist flexion crease. The subcutaneous fat is retracted, thereby exposing the superficial palmar fascia which is divided. The transverse carpal ligament is transected to the level of the distal wrist crease under direct vision; this forms the roof of the carpal tunnel. The antebrachial fascia is also divided. After ensuring good haemostasis the skin is closed; no deep sutures are required. Dressings are applied and a splint is applied to the wrist; this is done by keeping the elbow slightly flexed and keeping the wrist in a neutral position. Wrist splinting reduces the risk of anterior displacement of the median nerve and bowstringing of flexor tendons.

No scalpel vasectomy

No scalpel vasectomy (NSV) is considered a permanent method of sterilisation; it is the preferred procedure because it has a lower failure rate when compared to sutures or clip ligation. NSV is offered by a small number of general practitioners.

Patients undergoing NSV should be appropriately counselled about the risks and benefits of the procedure. Risks include vasovagal reaction, bleeding, haematoma formation, epididymal congestion, sperm granuloma formation, infection, acute and chronic post-operative pain, in addition to failure of the procedure. However, NSV is associated with a shorter operative time in addition to fewer complications when compared with traditional incisional techniques. Post-operative advice and post-procedure semen analysis to confirm azoospermia should also be discussed as part of pre-procedure counselling, so that informed consent can be taken.

Being able to palpate and mobilise the vasa deferentia is a pre-requisite for performing this procedure. Moreover, NSV may not be possible in the presence of large hydroceles or varicoceles. Scrotal scarring and scrotal infection are contraindications to the procedure.

The procedure

The patient is positioned in the supine position with the penis retracted upwards away from the operative field. The skin is cleaned with chlorhexidine and surgical drapes applied so that the scrotum is exposed.

The vas deferens (see *Fig. 7.1* for a reminder of male reproductive anatomy) is separated from the internal spermatic vessels and manipulated to a superficial position just below the middle scrotal raphe using a three-finger technique. The scrotal skin puncture site is anaesthetised. A perivasal block is achieved by injection of local anaesthetic along the course of the vas within the external spermatic fascial sheath, towards the inguinal ring. The vas deferens is fixed with ringed forceps. The scrotal skin and vas wall are pierced and dissected out using sharpened curved dissecting forceps. Using these instruments the vas deferens is delivered and the vasal sheath and vessels are then stripped from the vas. Once the vas has been delivered through the wound, both ends are occluded using electrocautery. After ensuring haemostasis, the occluded ends of the vas are returned into the scrotum.

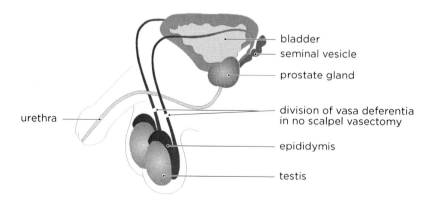

Figure 7.1: Male reproductive anatomy.

An identical procedure is performed for the opposite vas through the same puncture hole. No sutures are necessary for closure of the puncture hole; dressings are simply applied.

Post-operatively, the patient should be supine as much as possible for up to 48 hours, ice may be applied to the area and a scrotal support may be used. Patients are advised to seek medical attention if there is excessive bleeding, pain, swelling or discharge from the puncture site. Contraceptive cover is needed until azoospermia has been confirmed by semen sampling; the timing of these sample(s) may vary according to local guidance; however, azoospermia at 12 weeks is thought to predict long-term sterility.

Accreditation

Provision of NSV in general practice is reliant on having appropriate skills and being committed to ongoing continuing professional development[1]. Furthermore, an awareness of which cases would not be appropriate for NSV in a general practice setting is important. Moreover, contraceptive and sexual health issues need to be considered.

A Certificate in Local Anaesthetic Vasectomy from the FSRH of the RCOG may be obtained to demonstrate accreditation. In order to attain this, a minimum of 15 procedures should be observed by an approved trainer if there has been no prior vasectomy surgical experience, or a minimum of six procedures should be observed by an approved trainer if there is prior surgical experience of vasectomy. Assessment includes at least two Objective Structured Assessments of Skills, at least one Clinical Evaluation Exercise (mini-CEX), and at least one Case-Based Discussion (CbD). The FSRH advises that those performing NSV should have at least one operating list per month and perform 40 operations per year as a minimum. Moreover, audits should be undertaken to monitor complications, including failure rates.

Gynaecological procedures

A one-stop approach in a community setting for women with gynaecological problems may be developed if appropriate training and governance is in place. There is a GP with a Special Interest (GPwSI)-led primary care gynaecology service at NHS Bradford and Airedale which was estab-

---

[1] For further information refer to the British Association of No Scalpel Vasectomists (BANSV): www.aspc-uk.net/BANSV.htm [last accessed 9/1/2013]

lished in 2000 initially to reduce referrals to secondary care. This includes a one-stop diagnostic and treatment service, including resection of small endometrial polyps and fibroids, removal of 'lost' IUDs and insertion of Mirena®. Outpatient endometrial ablation under local anaesthesia may also be offered. Bradford University offers postgraduate education and accreditation to facilitate the above.

References

Bellamy N, Campbell J, Robinson V, Gee T, Bourne R & Wells G (2005) Intraarticular corticosteroid for treatment of osteoarthritis of the knee. *Cochrane Database Syst. Rev.* **2**:CD005328.

Cardone DA & Tallia AF (2002) Joint and soft tissue injection. *Am. Fam. Physician,* **66**: 283–8.

Coombes BK, Bisset L & Vicenzino B (2010) Efficacy and safety of corticosteroid injections and other injections for management of tendinopathy: a systematic review of randomised controlled trials. *Lancet,* **376**: 1751–67.

Creamer P (1997) Intra-articular corticosteroid injections in osteoarthritis: do they work and if so, how? *Ann. Rheum. Dis.* **56**: 634–6.

Genovese MC (1998) Joint and soft-tissue injection. A useful adjuvant to systemic and local treatment. *Postgrad. Med.* **103**: 125–34.

Schumacher HR (2003) Aspiration and injection therapies for joints. *Arthritis Rheum.* **49**: 413–20.

Stephens MB, Beutler AI & O'Connor FG (2008) Musculoskeletal injections: a review of the evidence. *Am. Fam. Physician,* **78**: 971–6.

Uthman I, Raynauld JP & Haraoui B (2003) Intra-articular therapy in osteoarthritis. *Postgrad. Med. J.* **79**: 449–53.

Further reading

Bell AD & Conaway D (2005) Corticosteroid injections for painful shoulders. *Int. J. Clin. Pract.* **59**: 1178–86.

Cardone DA & Tallia AF (2002) Diagnostic and therapeutic injection of the elbow region. *Am. Fam. Physician,* **66**: 2097–100.

Cardone DA & Tallia AF (2003) Diagnostic and therapeutic injection of the hip and knee. *Am. Fam. Physician,* **67**: 2147–52.

Department of Health (2007) *Guidance and competencies for the provision of services using GPs with Special Interests (GPwSIs). Dermatology and skin surgery.*

Finn L & Crook S (1998) Minor surgery in general practice – setting the standards. *Public Health Med.* **20**: 169–74.

Gaujoux-Viala C, Dougados M & Gossec L (2009) Efficacy and safety of steroid injections for shoulder and elbow tendonitis: a meta-analysis of randomised controlled trials. *Ann. Rheum. Dis.* **68**: 1843–9.

NICE (2006) *Improving outcomes for people with skin tumours including melanoma: the manual.*

NICE (2010) *Improving outcomes for people with skin tumours including melanoma (update): the management of low-risk basal cell carcinomas in the community.*

Shah N & Lewis M (2007) Shoulder adhesive capsulitis: systematic review of randomised trials using multiple corticosteroid injections. *Br. J. Gen. Pract.* **57**: 662–7.

Shin EK & Osterman AL (2008) Treatment of thumb metacarpophalangeal and interphalangeal joint arthritis. *Hand Clin.* **24**: 251–61.

Stainforth J & Goodfield MJ (1992) Cost-effectiveness of minor surgery in general practice. *Br. J. Gen. Pract.* **42**: 302–3.

Tallia AF & Cardone DA (2003) Diagnostic and therapeutic injection of the wrist and hand region. *Am. Fam. Physician,* **67**: 745–50.

Tallia AF & Cardone DA (2003) Diagnostic and therapeutic injection of the shoulder region. *Am. Fam. Physician,* **67**: 1271–8.

Yao J & Park MJ (2008) Early treatment of degenerative arthritis of the thumb carpometacarpal joint. *Hand Clin.* **24**: 251–61.

APPENDIX 1

Consent to minor surgery form

Patient agreement to investigation or treatment

Patient details (or pre-printed label)
Patient's surname / family name...
Patient's first names..
Date of birth...
Responsible health professional ....
Job title..
NHS number (or other identifier)...
☐ Male ☐ Female
Special requirements...
(e.g. other language / other communication method)

To be retained in patient's notes

Patient identifier/label

Name of proposed procedure or course of treatment
(include brief explanation if medical term not clear)

....

....

....

Statement of health professional
(to be filled in by health professional with appropriate knowledge of proposed procedure,
as specified in consent policy)

I have explained the procedure to the patient. In particular, I have explained:

The intended benefits .... *Removal of lesion, relief of symptoms,* ....
.... *diagnosis of lesion* ....

Serious or frequently occurring risks.... *Pain, bleeding, scarring, wound* ....
.... *infection / breakdown, need for further treatment or referral* ....
.... *to hospital, damage to nerves / blood vessels, reaction to local* ....
.... *anaesthesia* ....

Any extra procedures which may become necessary during the procedure

I have also discussed what the procedure is likely to involve, the benefits and
risks of any available alternative treatments (including no treatment) and any
particular concerns of this patient.

☐ The following leaflet/tape has been provided ....
.... *Minor surgery information leaflet* ....

This procedure will involve:.... *local anaesthesia* .... **(LA)**

Signature .... Date ....

Name (PRINT).. Job title.....................

Contact details ....
(if patient wishes to discuss options later)

Statement of interpreter *(where appropriate)*

I have interpreted the information above to the patient to the best of my ability and in a way in which I believe s/he can understand.

Interpreter's signature.. Date ....

Name (PRINT)..

Top copy accepted by patient: **yes / no**   *(please circle)*

Statement of patient

Please read this form carefully. If your treatment has been planned in advance, you should already have your own copy of page 2 which describes the benefits and risks of the proposed treatment. If not, you will be offered a copy now. If you have any further questions, do ask – we are here to help you. You have the right to change your mind at any time, including after you have signed this form.

I agree to the procedure or course of treatment described on this form.

I understand that you cannot give me a guarantee that a particular person will perform the procedure. The person will, however, have appropriate experience.

I understand that I will have the opportunity to discuss the details of anaesthesia with an anaesthetist before the procedure, unless the urgency of my situation prevents this. (This only applies to patients having general or regional anaesthesia.)

I understand that any procedure in addition to those described on this form will only be carried out if it is necessary to save my life or to prevent serious harm to my health.

I have been told about additional procedures which may become necessary during my treatment. I have listed below any procedures **which I do not wish to be carried out** without further discussion.

....

....

....

Patient's signature .... Date ....

Name (PRINT)..

A witness should sign below if the patient is unable to sign but has indicated his or her consent. Young people/children may also like a parent to sign here (see notes).

Signature .... Date ....

Name (PRINT)...

Confirmation of consent

(to be completed by a health professional when the patient is admitted for the procedure,
if the patient has signed the form in advance)

On behalf of the team treating the patient, I have confirmed with the patient that s/he has no further questions and wishes the procedure to go ahead.

Signature .... Date ....

Name (PRINT)... Job title..

Important notes: *(tick if applicable)*

☐   See also advance directive / living will (e.g. Jehovah's Witness form)

☐   Patient has withdrawn consent (ask patient to sign / date here)

APPENDIX 2

Patient information leaflet

Minor Surgery

Once your GP refers you for a minor surgical procedure you will be invited to attend a pre-assessment clinic for the doctor to assess your condition. You will be asked to give your consent for the procedure to be carried out.

On the day of your procedure you will be asked to sit or lie on a couch. The doctor will clean and prepare the skin. A local anaesthetic will be placed around the area to be operated on so that you will not be able to feel any pain during the procedure. The anaesthetic will take around 2 hours to wear off after the procedure.

Any skin lesion that is removed will be sent to the laboratory for close examination, and the results will be available around 2 weeks after the procedure.

If you have stitches, you will be given a follow-up appointment for their removal.

Your doctor will advise you at the time of your operation of any other care you may need to give your wound.

You will have a small scar – this may fade in time.

If you have any concerns about your procedure, please ask the doctor at your pre-assessment clinic appointment.

We recommend you wear loose-fitting clothes on the day of your operation.

APPENDIX 3

Consent to insertion of contraceptive implant form

Patient agreement to investigation or treatment

Patient details (or pre-printed label)

Patient's surname / family name ....

Patient's first names ....

Date of birth ....

Responsible health professional ....

Job title ....

NHS number (or other identifier) ....

☐ Male   ☐ Female

Special requirements ....
(e.g. other language / other communication method)

To be retained in patient's notes

Name of proposed procedure or course of treatment

(include brief explanation if medical term not clear)

....*Nexplanon Insertion*..................................

....

....

Statement of health professional

(to be filled in by health professional with appropriate knowledge of proposed procedure,
as specified in consent policy)

I have explained the procedure to the patient. In particular, I have explained:

The intended benefits ....*To prevent pregnancy*..

....

Serious or frequently occurring risks....*Allergic reaction to local*......................
....*anaesthesia, pain, bleeding, bruising, scarring, wound*......................
....*infection / breakdown, need for further treatment or referral to*..........
....*hospital, damage to nerves / blood vessels, migration of implant*......
....*irregular bleeding, hormonal side-effects, ovarian cysts*......................
....*failure rate (< 1%)*..

Any extra procedures which may become necessary during the procedure

I have also discussed what the procedure is likely to involve, the benefits and risks of any available alternative treatments (including no treatment) and any particular concerns of this patient.

☐   The following leaflet/tape has been provided ....
..........................*Long Acting Reversible Contraceptives*...............................

This procedure will involve:....*local anaesthesia*............ **(LA)**

Signature .... Date.......................................

Name (PRINT)... Job title..............................

Contact details ....
(if patient wishes to discuss options later)

Statement of interpreter *(where appropriate)*

I have interpreted the information above to the patient to the best of my ability and in a way in which I believe s/he can understand.

Interpreter's signature... Date ....

Name (PRINT)..

Top copy accepted by patient: **yes / no**   *(please circle)*

Statement of patient

Please read this form carefully. If your treatment has been planned in advance, you should already have your own copy of page 2 which describes the benefits and risks of the proposed treatment. If not, you will be offered a copy now. If you have any further questions, do ask – we are here to help you. You have the right to change your mind at any time, including after you have signed this form.

I agree to the procedure or course of treatment described on this form.

I understand that you cannot give me a guarantee that a particular person will perform the procedure. The person will, however, have appropriate experience.

I understand that I will have the opportunity to discuss the details of anaesthesia with an anaesthetist before the procedure, unless the urgency of my situation prevents this. (This only applies to patients having general or regional anaesthesia.)

I understand that any procedure in addition to those described on this form will only be carried out if it is necessary to save my life or to prevent serious harm to my health.

I have been told about additional procedures which may become necessary during my treatment. I have listed below any procedures **which I do not wish to be carried out** without further discussion.

....

....

....

Patient's signature... Date..

Name (PRINT)..

A witness should sign below if the patient is unable to sign but has indicated his or her consent. Young people / children may also like a parent to sign here (see notes).

Signature .... Date ....

Name (PRINT) ....

Confirmation of consent

(to be completed by a health professional when the patient is admitted for the procedure, if the patient has signed the form in advance)

On behalf of the team treating the patient, I have confirmed with the patient that s/he has no further questions and wishes the procedure to go ahead.

Signature .... Date ....

Name (PRINT) .... Job title ....

Important notes: (tick if applicable)

☐ See also advance directive / living will (e.g. Jehovah's Witness form)

☐ Patient has withdrawn consent (ask patient to sign / date here)

Index